The Undeniable TRUTH About FOOD

A PHASES approach to making CHANGES
that make a REAL difference to YOU and the PLANET

By Kylie Floate

BSc. (Nutrition) Grad.Dip.Ed (ECS)

Strategic Book Publishing and Rights Co.

Strategic Book Publishing and Rights Co.
12620 FM 1960, Suite A4-507
Houston, TX 77065
www.sbpra.com

ISBN: 978-1-61204-969-4

Book Design: Suzanne Kelly

*Dedicated to my four beautiful children
and The Golden Space™
for inspiring me to be all I can be.*

Contents

Introduction

As a young adult I was no different than any other person, I loved to eat fast food and lots of treats. I think it is part of having that initial freedom. Cutting those apron strings and buying whatever you like is liberating! If only the party could last forever....

When I first started studying nutrition I was a single mum and on a very tight budget. A typical meal was pasta and sauce or eggs on toast. Meat was a luxury I had twice per week and I never ate fruit. Even though I liked fruit, I saw it as an added expense. The few vegetables I did eat were the least expensive, with very little variety.

Changing my eating habits was not an easy step. I couldn't be a hypocrite. I had to put into practice what I was learning at university. So I took up gardening. I found that I could grow more than I needed for next to nothing. My daughter and I really bonded over our garden and I found she was much more likely to try something new when she had tended to the plant so lovingly.

I thought I had adopted fairly healthy eating habits. It wasn't perfect; we still had an ice-cream after swimming lessons and hot chips once a week. However, I absolutely believed that we followed a healthy diet.

When my daughter was eight I learned that she was very intolerant to certain food additives in seemingly healthy foods like bread, yoghurt and fruit juice. I had learned about food additives at university but for some reason I never made the connection. It took months of testing with a paediatrician to find out what was causing her severe eczema and volatile behaviour. And so our journey into the removal of food additives and other environmental toxins began.

My quest to help my daughter, lead me to the shocking truths about our food supply. I learnt about the disturbing number of pesticides and fertilisers that are used in agriculture. I also discovered that most produce is harvested when it is far from the realms of ripeness and placed in atmospheric controlled facilities. Months or sometimes years later, the so-called fresh produce is treated with artificial ripening agents that impact considerably on the taste, texture and health of the consumer.

The most disturbing fact was that we in Australia, the lucky country, have one the worst and most expensive food supplies in the world. It's disappointing to know that other governments have banned particular food additives as they have been proven to cause adverse effects, yet are still permitted for use in Australia.

Food preservation techniques have become down right Frankenstein in their approach and the meat industry has sunk to new lows in their practices.

Labelling laws allow sneaky, deceptive marketing, which takes advantage of consumer ignorance. Consumers who try to make a concerted effort to be healthy are frequently sabotaged by the 5% labelling loophole—a law that allows anything contained in the food item that is less than 5% of the overall product to be omitted from the label.

Furthermore, we now have a culture where highly acidic diets, derived from animal products and highly processed plant foods are causing chronic diseases such as osteoporosis, type two diabetes, cardiovascular disease and neurological disorders. The 'Western Diet' is literally killing us.

The media can be very confusing when it comes to healthy eating and in particular to losing weight. This book aims to sift through what is fact and useful knowledge and what are clever marketing schemes.

The information contained in this book came to me over a period of ten years. In fact, much of the information came to me in my first semester of university. At the age of twenty-three I wasn't ready to take much seriously. Change and taking onboard new concepts is something that has to occur progressively, when the time is right.

Food is a very personal part of our lives, most of us love food and making changes to that relationship is something not to be taken lightly. It's like quitting smoking, we all know that smoking is unhealthy, but apparently not all people are inspired to stop based on that knowledge alone. Timing is everything.

The book is divided into phases, as this is how I came to implement the knowledge and changes. It is unrealistic to radically change your lifestyle overnight and for it to be sustainable. It is important to take one step at a time; otherwise it just becomes a fad that doesn't last.

It will feel natural to progress to the next phase. If at anytime it feels forced or if what you're attempting to do doesn't resonate with you, revert back to the previous phase, there is no rush. Some people may never progress past phases one, two or three and that is really okay. We all have our own paths to follow. Most of us would agree that the Tibetan monks are among the most enlightened and peaceful people on Earth, but not all of us find the idea of meditating by a mountain all day that appealing.

My hope is that each person advances to at least phase three. The implications this would have on the global food supply would be significant. My greatest desire for our planet is a food supply that is produced with integrity, the way nature intended.

Multi-national corporations who produce our food are only concerned about making a profit. The more people who choose products that are produced with the consumer's health in mind, will provoke the other companies to change their ways. After all, the consumers are actually the ones who hold the power; no corporation wishes to be cut out of the marketplace. Use your shopping dollars wisely; think of it as voting each time you shop.

Phase One—Getting Healthy

No More Excuses

There has never been a better time in your life to embark on this transformational journey. We are all tired, we are all busy and we all have a million excuses as to why we can't make positive changes in our lives today. Procrastination is easy to fall prey to. We all do it. How many times have you tried to lose weight or start an exercise regime, or maybe you tried quitting smoking or drinking alcohol? We all have good intentions. Let's really do it this time.

It might be easier for some than others. Ask your family for support. Success is easier to attain when you include your family. I remember when my sister-in-law and I both had babies at almost the same time and we were trying to lose weight together. I had no one trying to sabotage my efforts, as I was a single mother. My sister-in-law on the other hand, had to contend with my brother who was constantly bringing home tubs of ice-cream or booking surprise restaurants meals. My brother thought he was being charming. Explain to your family that these changes are important to you; they might just surprise you!

Understanding Metabolism

The primary objective of the human body is to achieve homeostasis. Homeostasis is what the body regards as optimum. In order to assess the situation, the body is constantly under surveillance via a feedback system. This feedback system tells the brain if something in the body needs more of something or less of something. For example, if the core temperature of the body is too hot, the brain will initiate vasodilatation of the skin and induce sweating in order to cool the body down. It is very rare that the body is satisfied with its homeostatic state.

Metabolism is the speed at which the body gets all its jobs done. There are several factors that can affect the rate of metabolism. Illness will usually cause the metabolism rate to increase. Fatigue will cause the metabolism rate to slow down. Starvation mode, which can be triggered after not eating for as little as five hours, will cause an average decrease in the rate of metabolism of about 15%. Once starvation mode has been triggered it can be difficult to switch off, as the body needs convincing that the danger period is over—it is trying to keep you alive after all!

Menstruation and the few days prior (PMS), the rate of metabolism increases, requiring a woman to consume an extra 800 kilojoules (kJ) or 191 calories (cal) per day, hence the cravings!

Everyone knows someone who has a 'fast metabolism'. You know the person who can eat like a horse and never gain weight. This does tend to be genetic. Unfortunately, that means that some people are cursed with a genetically slow rate of metabolism. It doesn't have to be a life sentence; you can increase your rate of metabolism. The most effective way to achieve this is by increasing muscle mass by engaging in weight bearing exercise. The more cells the body has to service, the more energy it requires and the faster it will go!

If you think of your body as a car, the food is the fuel, the internal organs are the mechanics and the metabolism is the speed and efficiency of the car. If you put the correct fuel in the car, take it out of the driveway and have the car serviced regularly; the car going to run well and be less inclined to breakdown. Your body would like the same kind of treatment!

Energy Pathways

The human body can utilise energy from four different sources; carbohydrates, fat, protein and alcohol.

Carbohydrates yield 17kJ or 4cal per 100g.
Fat yields 37kJ or 8.8cal per 100g.
Protein yields 16kJ or 3.8cal per 100g.
Alcohol yields 28kJ or 6.6cal per 100g.

Kilojoules and calories are units of measurement to determine how much energy is inside food or drink. Kilojoules are used in countries that are working with the metric system and the term calories are used in countries aligned with the imperial system. They both measure energy in same way, by literally blowing up a food. The difference is in the measurement of heat. Kilojoules are measured by degrees centigrade; whereas calories are measured by degrees Fahrenheit. For each degree of temperature created in the explosion, it equates to one kilojoule or calorie. This is why water has zero kilojoules or calories, as you can't blow up water!

There is a lot of debate over the accuracy of this method, as it doesn't substantiate how much energy the body can access. It is also difficult to measure potential energy, as it is such an abstract concept. In addition, the body doesn't create an explosion to extract energy from food. The body uses hydrochloric acid to digest the food, which is then absorbed by the blood stream after the liver has converted the digested food into glucose molecules. The digestion process itself uses a lot of energy. This energy is called the basal metabolic rate; the energy required to breathe and exist without exerting additional energy to do anything else.

It is important to note that all food and drink sources (except water) are converted to glucose molecules. A common misconception is that fat is metabolised differently to sugar. It isn't. All food is broken down in to glucose; any excess glucose is converted to fat for storage. Fat doesn't get to bypass the process. Just as sugar is not incapable of being stored as fat! It always makes me laugh when I see lollies (candy) labelled as 99% fat free, giving the purchaser the impression that they won't cause weight gain!

The equation energy in – energy out = body weight is reality. It doesn't matter where the food comes from; fat, carbohydrates, protein or alcohol; if too much is consumed, it will be stored as fat.

Carbohydrates should make up 55% of the overall food intake. It comes from plant matter and can be either simple or complex. Simple carbohydrates refer to those already processed for example white table sugar. There is no challenge for the body to digest simple carbohydrates and usually results in a massive spike in the blood sugar levels. Complex carbohydrates, are just that, complex. They are a challenge for the body to break down and usually come with fibre that further assists digestion and stabilises blood sugar levels. Food sources include fruit, vegetables and grains. Carbohydrates are the only energy source, which can adequately nourish the brain. The brain can utilise protein if it is forced to, but the result is inferior and produces keytone bodies, which induces a poisoned acidic state.

Protein should contribute to 15% of the overall energy intake and comes from two sources—haem and non-haem, in other words plant or animals. Haem protein (animal derived) is the most bio-available as the body doesn't need to work hard to access the nutrients, like iron. Food sources include meat and dairy products. Non-haem protein is not inferior, the body just has to work harder to utilise the nutrients and they may not be as easily absorbed as the haem variety.

Fats are classified as four types; saturated, mono-unsaturated, poly-unsaturated and trans-fatty acids. Saturated fats come from animal sources and should not make up more than 7% of the recommended daily intake. Saturated fat contains high levels of LDL (low density, unhealthy) cholesterol. LDL cholesterol is considered bad as the body has a limited number of receptors to absorb cholesterol. If you think of the cholesterol as baseballs and the receptors as catcher's gloves. If there are too many cholesterol balls coming in and there are not enough receptors to 'catch' them, the balls are dropped. The cholesterol then burrows underneath the receptor and accumulates under the arterial walls. The cholesterol is attacked by free radicals, which turn the cholesterol rancid, forming an oozing substance. The pressure builds until a pimple or boil like structure forms, eventually bursting and depositing on the artery surface. This substance is known as plaque and continues to build until a blockage occurs, causing a myocardial infarction (heart attack).

Saturated fat is contained in meat, dairy and most 'junk' food. Cholesterol has an important function in hormones and cell membrane formation. However, the body would prefer to use HDL (high density) cholesterol, which is found in plant-based oils, grains, nuts and fish. A word on coconut oil (Palmatic oil), it contains 90% saturated fat, but legally can be labelled as a vegetable oil. Palmatic oil is cheap and provides a delicious flavour. It is often used in biscuits (cookies), cakes and cooking sauces.

Mono-unsaturated fats should make up 15% of the overall intake. These fats while they are able to be utilised for energy, also play an important role in cell membrane function and hormone production. Food sources are plant based, such as nuts, seeds and avocado.

Poly-unsaturated fats should make up 10% of the recommended daily intake. These fats can also be used for energy but have a vital role in cell division, blood platelet clotting and immune processes. Food sources include fish, dairy, nuts and other plant sources.

Trans-fatty acids are originally a mono-unsaturated fat, but when subjected to high heat, usually in the frying process or hydrogenation, it mutates. The result is a substance that behaves as a saturated fat, although legally it can be classified as a mono-unsaturated fat. Fast foods are the biggest producers of trans-fat. Trans-fat should be avoided wherever possible.

The last type of energy that can be utilised is alcohol. Unfortunately, the by-product that is produced is methanal, which is the substance that causes a hangover. Regular alcohol consumption is the quickest way to over-consume energy and cause excess weight. Some drinks, particularly spirits that are mixed with a soft-drink (soda) and can equate to a meal, have a few of those a night and fat will be laid down very quickly! Obviously alcohol is an unhealthy, unnecessary substance that should not contribute to the recommended daily intake.

Calculating Your Estimated Energy Requirements (EER)

Now you know what proportions make up the recommended daily intake (RDI). Here's how to work out your personal estimated energy requirement.

Women Aged		
	15-22yrs	7900kJ or 1886cal
	23-50yrs	7500kJ or 1793cal
	51-65yrs	7100kJ or 1695cal

Based on a height of 162cm. For every centimetre you are above of below that height, add or subtract 105kJ or 25cal. If you need to convert your height from feet and inches into centimetres, there are 30.48cm in 1 foot and 2.54cm in an inch.

If you have a very physical job, you can add 2100kJ or 501cal. If you are breast-feeding you can add 1500kJ or 358cal. If you are very inactive and sit behind a desk all day, you can subtract 840kJ or 200cal.

Men Aged		
	15-22yrs	10900kJ or 2603cal
	23-50yrs	9600kJ or 2292cal
	51-65yrs	8400kJ or 2006cal

Follow the steps above. If you're wondering why men require more energy per day than women; it is because generally men have more muscle mass and more cells per surface area than women.

For example I am 34 and 168cm and I am active everyday, but I'm no labourer so my calculations will be:

$$105 \times 6 + 7500 = 8130kJ \text{ per day.}$$

When I multiply 8130 by 55% I get a carbohydrate requirement of 4471kJ

My protein requirement equals 1219kJ per day

My saturated fat requirement equals 406kJ per day

My monounsaturated fat requirement equals 1219kJ per day

My polyunsaturated fat requirement equals 813kJ per day

Another method to calculate your estimated energy requirements:

(0.034 x weight in kilograms + 3.538) x 1.5 (activity factor) x 1000 = Daily energy requirements in kilojoules. Note kilojoules can be converted to calories by multiplying the number by 0.24.

Energy factor can be varied according to different activity level.

Bed rest	1.2
Very sedentary	1.3
Sedentary	1.4
Light	1.5
Light/moderate	1.7
Moderate	1.8
Heavy	2.1
Very heavy	2.3

Most people would be classified as light. If you go for a daily walk and are on your feet most of the day you would be 'light/moderate'. A person who does a daily vigorous gym work out and is on their feet most of the day would be 'moderate'. Someone who does a physical job like building and construction would be classified as 'heavily active' and in order to be 'very heavy' one would need to be an elite athlete.

The 80/20 Rainbow Diet

The essence of what we are trying to achieve is 80% healthy food and 20% treat food. Unfortunately, the current culture is the exact reverse. This has come about mainly due to World War II and The Great Depression. You see people during this time really suffered. They were lucky to obtain sufficient food and the concept of indulgence was ridiculous. After the war and when the baby boomer generation came into being, the parents who had experienced such hardship, were determined to make their children's lives much brighter. Foods became richer and more abundant. Dessert became a regular occurrence. Fast food restaurants took flight and the incidence of obesity became more common. The concept of a treat became lost and everyday became like Christmas. It is understandable that this happened, but the war ended over sixty years ago. It is time to end the party. Just because we can indulge everyday, doesn't mean we should. The trouble is; it has become difficult to determine what constitutes a treat.

Food labelling has become so deceptive that unless you know how to read between the lines, it is easy to be led astray. How many people have bought a product labelled as 'lite', 'fat-free' or 'reduced fat' and thought it was the healthy option? In reality these products are usually loaded with sugar and more food additives, with marginally less energy (kJ) than the full fat variety! In Australia, the legislation is only clear for those products that claim to be 'low' in something. In order to be labelled as 'low fat' or 'low sugar', it must contain less than 3g of fat or sugar per 100g or less than 3% fat or sugar of the overall product. Be wary about what has been added to compensate for the taste.

Ideally, a product shouldn't contain more than 10g sugar per 100g or 10% of the overall product. Often the sugar is labelled as part of the carbohydrate content, making it impossible for the consumer to tell how much sugar has actually been added.

Total fat in a product should not exceed 8g per 100g or 8% of the overall product.

In real terms, the daily 20% treat food should look something like this: four plain sweet biscuits (cookies), like the milk arrowroot variety or two evil biscuits (chocolate coated cookies), a couple of scoops of ice cream or a small piece of cake. Better yet, choose snacks like fruit, small handful of nuts (don't over indulge as nuts are very energy dense), tub of yoghurt or low fat dip and veggie sticks.

If you choose to eat healthily most of the time, when it comes to special occasions, you can eat what you like. Eat properly all week then go out and enjoy a beautiful meal on the weekend. Meet a friend at a nice café and enjoy a decadent piece of cake. Enjoy your favourite chocolate bar or potato chips a couple of times per week. A healthy lifestyle is not about deprivation, it is about being realistic about what is reasonable to consume in a day.

The other 80% should contain a wide variety of fruits, vegetables, grains, lean meats, fish and nuts. Variety in the food intake equates to a greater selection of nutrients and phytochemicals. The body has a tall list of essential nutrients that are needed to function properly. Phytochemicals are wonderful compounds found in fruits and vegetables that have been found to exhibit anti-cancer and anti-ageing properties.

Studies have shown that people are creatures of habit and consume a diet of little variety. Be adventurous and try things that you may have previously disliked or never even tried. Did you know that taste sensation is the first of the senses to deplete? On average, a baby has 50,000 more taste buds than an adult. Unfortunately, childhood dislikes are often unnecessarily carried through to adulthood.

Be sure to enjoy special occasions. When we eat a healthy diet, it gives us the freedom to enjoy those special celebrations. Just remember special occasions aren't very special if they occur every day!

Breakfast

Breakfast is, as we all should know 'the most important meal of the day'. Research shows that those who skip breakfast have a decreased ability for attention and have slower metabolisms. Food and coffee are what most people think about upon waking, but what the body is really seeking is water. Unfortunately, the common occurrence is a sugary breakfast cereal; or butter laden toast; washed down with a cup of tea or coffee. Tea and coffee contains three ingredients that the body could do with out. First of all is phytates, which are also contained in wholegrain breakfast cereal, wholegrain toast and many other healthy food sources. However, phytates inhibit iron and calcium absorption. Tea and coffee also contains tannins that interfere with iron absorption. Like phytates, tannins are found in many healthy foods. The last ingredient is caffeine. Caffeine is just a drug and has no nutritional component, but does have a powerful effect on the body. Caffeine increases the heart rate making a person feel more alert and it also spares carbohydrate uptake making the available energy more efficient. Athletes use caffeine to great effect and doping levels are routinely tested. However it is a drug. I'm sure we could all perform with a little amphetamine use also, but it puts a strain on the body that is unnecessary. Coffee and tea serve no nutritional benefit and actually sabotage your efforts to be healthy. Coffee and tea is a part of our culture. If you find that eliminating these beverages altogether is too difficult, try to consume them two hours before or after food so that nutrient absorption is not interfered with.

Breakfast should contain complex carbohydrates, which are a challenge to digest, giving sustained energy and powerful brain fuel. Many breakfast cereals are highly processed which are easily broken down and cause a huge spike in blood sugar levels. Try to opt for a muesli or porridge. Oats contains a lot of soluble fibre and are a great way to start the day. Some of the compressed biscuits are okay, but the sugar content should never exceed 10g per 100g or 10% of the overall product. Try adding fresh fruit. Other ideas include yoghurt with fresh fruit and nuts or a delicious fruit smoothie.

In relation to milk, there are A1 and A2 varieties. Depending on the country, A1 will be the most common type available. However, A2 milk is the original type of milk that we drank for centuries and is the most easily digested by humans. A1 milk became more favourable to dairy farmers as the yield is significantly higher than that of A2 cows. Unfortunately, the quality of A1 milk is inferior and is difficult for many people to digest. Let's not forget that cows' milk in intended for cows, not humans. Cows' milk is high in phosphate, which decreases the bioavailability of calcium. Goats' milk is closer to human milk in terms of composition. There are also many milk alternatives available including oat, rice, soy and almond.

Lunch

I'm sure you've heard the wives tale that say you should eat breakfast as a king, lunch as a queen and dinner as a pauper. Well there is a lot of truth in that. Going by that rationale, lunch should be more substantial than the evening meal. This concept is easy in theory, but more difficult in practice. You see our lives are so diverse that what and how we eat at lunchtime is largely influenced by our occupation or lifestyle. Some people have the luxury of being at home or in an office, with cooking facilities available. Others are sat in their cars, eating on the go. Some less fortunate people must eat in restaurants with clients or colleagues as part of their job description.

If you are lucky enough to have cooking facilities at your disposal, then there really is no excuse. Make a nice salad or some lean meat or fish with vegetables.

For those who are stuck in their cars, get up ten minutes early and make a packed lunch. It is really all it takes. Alternatively, make a batch of soup on the weekend and take a thermos. Just whatever you do, avoid the drive through fast food outlet.

If your work situation requires table service, be smart with your selection. Avoid pasta, anything with a cream sauce, breadcrumbs, cheese and heavy dressings. Most restaurants will have something involving lean meat or fish with vegetables or salad on the menu. Always skip dessert, or choose a fruit platter and try to vary the cuisine if possible.

Dinner

The most important aspect of eating dinner is the timing. It is really important to consume dinner at least two hours before bedtime. During sleep the body is engaged in growth and repair. It doesn't like forfeiting any of its allotted time for digestion.

This can be achieved by ensuring that food is on hand to prepare shortly after getting home. Don't fill up on snacks and delay dinner. Have something in the freezer that can be pulled out when the temptation to call for take-away arises. Try to be organised.

If you have children endeavour to eat with them regularly. This may entail eating earlier, but when healthy eating habits are modelled to children, they are more likely to adopt these practices in later life. In order for children to maximise their growth and repair potential, they really need to eat by five or six o'clock, depending on the bedtime.

Some helpful guidelines:

- Limit pasta or rice to a maximum of twice per week.
- Select quality cuts of meat, as they are more nutrient dense. It is far better to eat meat less often and choose premium cuts, than eat meat everyday and select the lesser cuts.
- Limit red meat to twice per week, chicken twice per week and have the remaining three meals as fish or vegetarian.
- Include some raw food everyday, as many of the vitamins and minerals are destroyed in the cooking process.
- Limit potatoes to a maximum of three times per week, as they are energy dense and quite low in nutrients.
- Keep egg intake to a maximum of four per week, as they are hard for the body to digest and high in cholesterol.

The Serotonin Effect

Serotonin is an important neurotransmitter that produces feelings of well-being and is thought to facilitate sleep. It is the basis of many antidepressant medications such as *prozac*. These medications inhibit the reuptake of serotonin, leaving the 'flood gates' open and thereby allowing more circulating serum serotonin. In theory, this should make for happy people who sleep like babies. This effect can be created through food combinations instead of pharmacology.

There is an essential amino acid called tryptophan. It is classified as essential as the body must obtain it through food.

Tryptophan is found in a variety of foods, such as meat, eggs, soy, seeds (especially sesame), nuts, grains (such as wheat, quinoa and amaranth) and legumes. It is estimated that adults require 3.5g or 1.2oz of tryptophan per day.

The problem is, tryptophan has to compete with other amino acids for metabolism and needs very specific conditions to thrive. This is achieved by consuming a meal rich in tryptophan and then approximately half an hour later, eating something sweet that contains mostly carbohydrates. It is interesting that we have a culture that appreciates the concept of dessert! It is exciting to think that there is actually a scientific basis for eating dessert!

When we crave something sweet after a meal, it's important that we satisfy the body in order to produce optimal brain chemistry. However, this can be achieved the healthy or evil way. The healthy way is to choose fresh, dried or cooked fruit. The less desirable way is to eat ice-cream and pudding.

The Consequences of Obesity

The latest research indicates that one in two women and one in three men are overweight or obese. Subsequently, there is a profound prevalence of diabetes mellitus (type two, late on-set) and heart disease; including hypertension (high blood pressure), elevated blood serum cholesterol and myocardial infarction (heart attack).

Diabetes mellitus results when there is an accumulation of fat around the pancreas, preventing the release of insulin into the bloodstream. The role of insulin is to convert excess blood glucose (sugar) into glycogen for storage. When insulin is unable to perform its job, blood glucose levels remain high, until the excess glucose is eventually excreted in the urine. The complications that can occur include: lethargy, kidney disease/failure, blindness, loss of limbs (particularly toes), impaired fertility, neuropathy (loss of sensation), hyperglycaemic coma, heart disease and stroke. Abdominal fatness is the biggest risk factor in developing diabetes mellitus. In fact a person with a blood glucose reading of <8mmol/L can actually completely reverse the symptoms and avoid developing the disease by losing weight. When the disease has escalated to a blood glucose level of 12mmol/L it is usually too late, as the pancreas has malfunctioned and the only course of action is management. The prescription usually involves small frequent meals, which are high in fibre and thus have a low glycaemic index.

As previously discussed, high cholesterol is caused by the laying down of plaque in the arteries, which builds, causing a blockage in the flow of blood, otherwise known as a heart attack. Hypertension is usually caused by the building of plaque in the arteries, but can also be caused by a high sodium intake, which disturbs the electrolyte ratio, causing interference in electrical impulses in the body (particularly the heart).

Risk Assessment

There are several ways to determine your risk to these preventable diseases. The first method is the waist to hip ratio. This is determined by measuring the waist and hips with a sewing tape measure. Then using a calculator, divide the hip measurement into the waist measurement.

For example 88 cm (waist) ÷ 102 cm (hips) = 0.86

Or 34" (waist) ÷ 40" (hips) = 0.85

Women with a waist to hip ratio greater than 0.8 are considered at risk of disease.

Men with a waist to hip ratio greater than 0.9 are considered at risk of disease.

Another measure is the Body Mass Index (BMI). Only use this if you are of average height. Using a calculator divide your weight in kilograms by your height in metre^2.

For example $72 \div (1.68)^2 = 25.51$

Or weight in lbs ÷ (height in inches)^2 x 703 = BMI

For example $150 \div (66)^2 \times 703 = 24.20$

Healthy weight range is 22-26

The most reliable method is of course to perform a blood test. The blood glucose test involves taking two lots of blood one after fasting and one after consuming a sugary drink. The serum cholesterol involves the standard blood test. While you're at the doctors it is a good idea to have a basic physical. Health outcomes are drastically impacted by whether a condition is detected early or late. Unfortunately, men usually have the worst health outcomes as they notoriously leave it too late to make that appointment to get checked out. Most people know if they are carrying too much weight, or if something is not right.

Psychology of Food

Weight is merely a symptom or a manifestation of an underlying cause. If this cause is not addressed, weight is almost always regained and is why diets don't work! Most people fall into one of these four categories:

LEARNED BEHAVIOUR: Significant others, particularly family strongly shape who we are and how we behave. From the moment we are born we are being socialised, absorbing the actions being modelled by the people we spend the most time with. How we approach food is deeply entrenched in our upbringing. This doesn't have to be a life sentence. Awareness is the key to making changes. Take responsibility for your own life and choose a healthy lifestyle.

TIME MANAGEMENT: People are too busy to cook healthy foods. They have no time to read food labels and to investigate what they are actually eating. They have a tendency to buy pre-packaged or fast foods. Getting organised can be a challenge that extends far beyond eating habits. Sometimes it's hard to say no. It is easy to become over-committed. Trying to have it all and do it all is a tall order. Start with watching an hour less of television per week and really work at restructuring your life. Be prepared. If after school activities or peak hour traffic means getting home late, have a meal frozen ready to go. When you cook, make double, it takes less time and dishes overall than cooking every night. Leftovers can be frozen, or alternatively, there is no shame in eating the same meal two nights in a row—with four kids, I do this frequently!

EMOTIONAL ISSUES: People who eat to self medicate. They crave sugar highs; have low fibre diets that lead to brief satiation. They have a tendency to suffer from mood swings and will consume high-carb foods that give a *prozac* like effect. Eating equals happiness, de-stress or numbness. There's also this 'I deserve' mentality, where we reward ourselves with our favourite food for getting through a tiring day. Find an alternative way to soothe yourself. You do 'deserve', but surely there is something other than food that could bring a smile to your face!

IGNORANCE: Clever advertising easily influences many well-intentioned people. Lacking knowledge of how food is metabolised or what the bodily requirements are, can lead to poor food choices. It is also important to understand the need for sufficient physical exercise. Energy in minus energy out equals your body weight. Find out how much and of which types of food your body requires, stop eating for the sake of it or out of habit. Make simple brand changes that won't be noticed. Remember that treats are treats and everyday is not Christmas. Find out what is a treat and what is everyday food. Just because we are not living through war rations or The Great Depression, just because we can indulge, doesn't mean we should. Our parents and grandparents went without—we are over indulged. Start being realistic with what is reasonable to consume in a day!

Weight Loss

Weight loss is usually achieved by moving more and eating less! Studies have shown that exercise has more influence over weight loss and food intake is the greatest indicator of health and nutritional status. When diet and exercise join forces, weight loss is inevitable.

The first step is to reduce the energy intake by 2000kJ or 500cal. By doing so, it will create a negative nitrogen balance. A negative nitrogen balance indicates body mass loss and must be kept consistent in order to maximise weight loss. This is why yo-yo dieting is usually ineffective. If you're actively intending to lose weight, keep doing it until the desired results are achieved. Having good days and bad days in terms of food intake rarely leads to sustained weight loss. The body in its quest to maintain homeostasis has a set point of body mass it tries to maintain. If the body usually receives 10,000kJ or 2388cal per day it will function on the basis that this will continue. If suddenly the daily intake drops to 8,000kJ or 1910cal per day it will take some time for the body to accept this change as permanent. Yo-yo dieting only prolongs this process. Remember that severe food deprivation leads to starvation mode activation, causing a slowed metabolism, making it very difficult to lose weight.

The four-week diet that I discuss in detail later is a good tool for the body and psyche to adjust to a reduced energy intake. Another useful tool is keeping a food diary of everything that is consumed during an average week, including the times of day and the motivation for the consumption. Actively recognise when hunger sets in and what the body is craving. Try to identify habits and set about making resolutions for a new way of life.

Research shows that on average between the ages of 30 and 40 a person will gain 1-2kg or 2-4lbs each year, making the weight gain subtle, but resulting in a gain of 10-20kg or 20-40lbs during that time period. Additionally, when a person does lose weight most will regain the weight within two years. In order for weight loss to be permanent, authentic life changes must be made.

The current recommendation for exercise is 30-60 minutes of vigorous activity each day. This can involve anything, even sex; the key is to feel too out of breath to talk comfortably. When we have a reduced oxygen intake, the body will use glycogen, of which we have about 1-2 hours supply. The primary purpose of glycogen is for the fight or flight response. When the stores are depleted and the body has oxygen available once again; the body converts fat to glycogen at vacuum speed to replenish the muscle stores. The preferred energy source for daily activities is fat. The fat is broken down into glucose molecules at a slow steady rate. We must tap into those glycogen stores if we want to lose weight efficiently. Initially, this may involve a brisk walk or bike ride. As the level of fitness increases, you may be able to go for a run or take part in an aerobics class. We are all individuals and enjoy different activities. Choose something that is enjoyable to you. Remember the body likes to achieve homeostasis, so keep it guessing and mix it up a little. Varying exercise leads to faster weight loss.

High Protein and Detox Diets

A high protein diet is a very effective method to lose weight quickly. However, it is important to note that this diet it strictly for two weeks, as the body really does not appreciate it. High protein diets induce ketosis because the body is forced to utilise protein for energy. Ketosis is a poisoned acid state that places an enormous strain on the kidneys. In addition, when the brain is forced to accept keytone bodies in place of carbohydrates it negatively affects mental computation. A person is likely to be short-tempered, easily confused, and irrational, with a short attention span. It is fortunate that the human body is amazingly resilient and can cope with a two-week high protein diet without causing permanent damage. Just be sure to plan the high protein diet for a time that doesn't include important meetings, exams or during an already highly stressed situation. Most people lose about 10Kg or 20lbs over the 4-week period (that includes the coming two-week detox). How much weight you lose will depend on your start weight, metabolism and consistency.

The big no no's are alcohol, bread, pasta, rice and starchy vegetables (potatoes, pumpkin, corn).

2 week High Protein Guidelines

Breakfast choices: eggs, bacon, meat, seafood, smoothie. My pick is having a smoothie containing 3/4-cup cold skim milk, 1 cold banana, 1 teaspoon of hot chocolate powder and blended for about 30 seconds. You can use any fruit.

If you go for the bacon and eggs, be sure to have a piece of fruit about 1/2 hour later to induce the serotonin effect.

Morning Tea choices: yoghurt, fruit, a handful of nuts or small choc milk.

Lunch choices: meat and salad, tuna, eggs, cheese, seafood. Some people go and get a big hunk of ham. I suggest roasting a lump of meat that can be eaten over a few days with a little salad.

Afternoon tea: same as morning tea

Dinner choices: meat and vegetables/salad. This should be the easiest as it won't impact the rest of the family.

Dessert: jelly, stewed fruit, 1 scoop of ice cream or sorbet.

For morning or afternoon tea and dessert the portions should be small, for example 1/2-cup yoghurt. The other meals have as much as you like, most people have a limit to how much meat or eggs they can stomach. You will actually look forward to the meat free component of the detox-diet!

Consume at least a litre or 34floz of water. You can have tea or coffee, but no fruit juice.

Important—weigh and measure yourself before the commencement of the diet and then four weeks after the completion of the detox diet. This is because your body is actually a reflection of the conditions it experienced approximately four week prior. Hydration is the only factor that can influence this outcome. A person can survive about a week without food, but will only last three days without water. So if you're stranded in the desert and you have food but no water, consuming the food will actually kill you faster!

Make sure you engage in at least one hour of physical activity each day. Remember exercise has the most powerful influence over weight loss. Ensure there is an element of huff and puff. The body needs to be taken out of its comfort zone, even if it means walking up a steep hill, just do something that will challenge the body for at least part of the one hour of exercise.

During the two weeks of consuming a high protein diet, the body will accumulate a lot of toxins (not to mention the pre-existing toxins!) The detox diet is designed to help flush and purify the system. Like the high protein diet, the detox is not designed to go beyond the two week period, I wouldn't advise doing either of the diets more than twice per year.

Detox Guidelines

No red meat, fish is fine (eat it everyday if you want, make sure it's fresh and not canned or crumbed). A little chicken, with a maximum twice per week.

No Dairy, stick to yoghurt and dairy substitutes such as rice, oat or soymilk.

No Tea or Coffee, while the caffeine is of some concern, it's actually the phytates and tannins that we are trying to reduce, which interfere with nutrient absorption.

Limit Potato intake, the good news is you can have some root vegetables, but don't over indulge; try not to exceed one potato per day (even if they are in a soup).

No bread or flour based foods—we want whole foods that are a challenge for the body the breakdown and are loaded with nutrients (no empty calories).

No refined cereals—stick to the whole grains, like oats or muesli.

No pasta or white rice—some brown or wild rice is okay. You might like to try some grains like quinoa or couscous.

Limit egg intake—no more than one per day.

Do utilise nuts, particularly natural ones (not roasted) and buy sulphite free. Remember nuts are very energy dense so only one to two handfuls per day.

Do eat lots of fruit and vegetables of a wide variety—try to buy non-artificially ripened, pesticide free produce.

Eat legumes and pulses, they contain the amino acid methionine which very good for digestion.

Drink lots of water, aim for 2 litres or 68floz per day—small frequent sips is far kinder to the kidneys than guzzling half a litre at a time.

Breakfast suggestions

Fruit smoothie (For example: 1 cup of frozen berries and half a glass of apple juice blended).

Porridge or muesli made with a dairy alternative is a great start to the day. If you're going the smoothie option, be creative, there are lots of possibilities.

Morning Tea suggestions

1 cup of yoghurt.

Fruit or cut up veggies with hummus or tabouli

Handful of nuts.

Lunch suggestions

Make a pot of soup or a big salad with light vinaigrette (sulphite free).

You could have fish or chicken with steamed veggies or salad.

If you're forced to buy takeaway as I am when I have to go to the city Nando's chicken salad is a good option, or a subway salad bowl.

Afternoon Tea

Same as morning tea

Dinner

Fish or chicken with vegetables or salad (you can have fish every night if you want, but limit chicken to twice a week).

Veggie and lentil patties are always a hit in my house; just roll them in quinoa or couscous instead of breadcrumbs.

Chicken and vegetable stir fry with some rice, quinoa or couscous.

Soup, all varieties, but no cream. Try blending ½ cup of any nut variety with a cup of water for five minutes, it makes for a great cream substitute and tastes amazing!

Dessert

Fruit—try something decadent like a mango, strawberries, pineapple or dragon fruit.

Dried fruit—I love those pawpaw spears. Remember dried fruit is very energy dense, so just a small handful.

Two scoops of sorbet

Remember not to eat two hours before your bedtime!

Have a glass of water upon waking.

Weight Loss Tips for Maintenance

- 80/20 ratio exercise flexible restraint (i.e. 80% good food, 20% treat).
- Don't buy foods you have no will power for.
- No shopping on an empty stomach.
- Don't skip meals, eat every 3 hours.
- Make sure there is a variety of good food to choose from.
- One hour of exercise per day, including vigorous exercise at least three times per week.
- Limit of two slices of wholegrain bread per day.
- Limit pasta or rice dishes to three times per week.
- All fat yields the same amount energy (kJ).
- Energy in—energy out = weight.
- Don't mistake thirst for hunger, always have a drink first.
- Counting kilojoules for a few days may be useful for you to determine eating habits but don't do it long term.
- Be realistic you will see visible results, other than hydration, you generally are a reflection of your lifestyle four weeks ago.
- Chew food thoroughly, savour each mouthful.
- Opt for wholemeal as it aids digestion and energy is released slower, making you feel fuller for longer.
- Seaweed contains all the elements in nature try adding it to meals.
- The less water a food contains the more energy it contains.
- Don't be a slave to the scales, weigh yourself once per month in the morning, before breakfast after a bowel movement.
- Have meals frozen to deter from buying takeaway.

- Have a healthy mental attitude to weight loss, believe that you can do it. Obsession is not healthy.
- Changing old habits can be disorientating, be patient, a four week plan is a good tool to alter a lifestyle permanently.
- Alcohol contains more energy than carbohydrates, plus any additional sugar in the mixer, a couple of drinks can easily equate to a meal.
- Don't eat two hours before sleep.
- Try using a pedometer and aim for 10,000 steps per day.
- Reconsider seconds wait twenty minutes. It takes this long for your brain to register that you have eaten—have a glass of water instead.
- Recognise emotional eating and choose another way to cope: go for a walk, listen to music, make a phone call, clean the house, have a drink.
- Brush teeth after eating to deter grazing.

Fibre

Fibre is a fabulous substance that is contained in plant-derived foods. There are two types of fibre, soluble and insoluble. Soluble fibre usually refers to the resistance starch found within the plant. Insoluble fibre refers to the outer husks or skins of fruits, vegetables, nuts and cereals.

The function of insoluble fibre is to give poo its bulk and attract water, thereby increasing transit time. When poo is able to have extended contact with the cells lining the colon, toxins can pass through the cell wall. In addition, butyric acid, which is produced by dietary fibre, provides metabolic energy to the cells of the colon, making them healthy and inhibiting the growth of cancerous cells. Insufficient insoluble fibre is believed to be the leading cause of bowel cancer.

Soluble fibre slows down the release of sugar from carbo-hydrates, preventing a spike in blood glucose levels. This action results in a sustained release of energy, making a person feel fuller for longer. The use of soluble fibre is particularly beneficial in the prevention and treatment of diabetes. Soluble fibre also has a positive effect on serum cholesterol levels by facilitating its excretion. In the absence of soluble fibre, cholesterol is more likely to by re-absorbed, creating higher levels of blood serum cholesterol. Therefore the use of soluble fibre is of particular importance to those with high blood pressure and heart disease.

The recommended daily intake of dietary fibre is 30g or 1oz. A healthy diet should provide sufficient fibre, but a fibre supplement may also be beneficial.

Vitamins, Minerals and Supplements

Vitamins and minerals are vital for bodily function. If a person consumes a healthy balanced diet, there is no need for supplements. There seems to be a dangerous overuse of vitamin and mineral supplements. First of all there's seems to be a school of thought that believes a normal intake of vitamin and minerals is good, so a high intake must be better. This is a dangerous attitude as many of the vitamins and minerals have toxicity levels or have 'rebound' effects. Rebound effects are when the body gets used to a high level of supplementation and when the intake is stopped suddenly, deficiency symptoms are induced, even if the dietary intake was already adequate. High vitamin and mineral intake has no purpose, as most have very little potential for storage and therefore must be excreted. Hence the fluorescent yellow urine; otherwise know as very expensive wee.

This section will examine each vitamin and mineral in turn and including its function, deficiency, toxicity, food sources and recommended daily intake (RDI).

Vitamin A

Function: essential for vision, bone formation and skin.

Deficiency: dry mucous membranes, poor night vision, blindness, decreased appetite and lack of immunity. It is the leading cause of blindness in third world countries.

Toxicity: Yellowing of the skin and associated with lung cancer.

Food Sources: Animal sources in the form of retinol include meat and dairy. Plant sources in the form of beta-carotene include apricots, peaches, mangoes, rockmelon, carrots, sweet potato, pumpkin, parsley, broccoli and spinach.

RDI: 750µg (retinol equivalents)

Vitamin B1 Thiamin

Function: involved in carbohydrate metabolism, digestion, heart and nerve function.

Deficiency: occurs after a short period of time, as there is a limited storage capacity within the body. Symptoms include: lethargy and in severe cases, Berri Berri. Berri Berri is a condition that affects the nervous system and heart. Can also manifest psychosis. Deficiency is usually associated with alcoholism and a poor diet.

Toxicity: no known effects.

Food Sources: nuts, seeds, legumes, soybeans yeast, whole-grains and bread. Thiamin is lost during the cooking process, particularly boiling.

RDI: 1.1mg/day

Vitamin B2 Riboflavin

Function: cell respiration and energy metabolism.

Deficiency: visual disturbances, tongue inflammation, dry cracked lips and cracks in the corner of the mouth. There is very little storage capacity for riboflavin.

Toxicity: no known effects in adults. Infants can fail to thrive.

Food Sources: dairy, eggs, yeast, almonds, soybeans, chives, parsley, spinach and broccoli. Riboflavin is very sensitive to cooking, light and alkaline conditions.

RDI: 1.4mg/day

Vitamin B3 Niacin

Function: involved in the metabolism of energy and essential for growth and repair.

Deficiency: loss of appetite, weakness, stomach cramps, pellagra dermatitis and dementia.

Toxicity: large doses from supplements can cause nausea, skin rashes and liver and heart damage.

Food Sources: meat, peanuts, sesame seeds, potatoes, peas, mushrooms, dried fruits and yeast.

RDI: 1.6mg/day

Vitamin B4 Pantothenic Acid

Function: energy metabolism; involved in the formation of haemoglobin and neurotransmitters; as well as the synthesis of amino acids, fatty acids, steroid hormones and vitamin D.

Deficiency: has never been reported.

Toxicity: no known effects.

Food Sources: widely distributed in plant and animal foods. Intestinal bacteria are also able to synthesise B4. However, does lose up to 50% during the cooking process and is sensitive to acid and alkaline conditions.

RDI: none set in Australia. USA has set 4-7mg/day

Vitamin B5 Biotin

Function: a co-enzyme in many processes; including: formation of red blood cells and the synthesis and metabolism of proteins such as serotonin.

Deficiency: no know effects.

Toxicity: no known toxicity, but prolonged use can cause dependency.

Food Sources: soybeans, eggs, fish, wholemeal bread; trace amounts occur in most fruit and vegetables. Significant amounts of B5 are produced by intestinal bacteria. B5 is sensitive to air, oxygen and alkaline conditions.

RDI: none set in Australia. USA has set 100-200mg/day.

Vitamin B6 Pyridoxine

Function: energy release, protein metabolism and the synthesis and metabolism of serotonin.

Deficiency: irritability, mental depression, abnormal brainwaves, impaired conduction of nerve impulses, convulsive seizures and immune deficiency.

Toxicity: regular and prolonged use of supplements may lead to dependency and loss of sensation. B6 is often prescribed to relieve premenstrual syndrome, but there is very limited evidence of its effectiveness.

Food Sources: widely distributed in plant and animal food. Particularly good sources include: walnuts, bananas, legumes, nuts, potatoes, meat, fish and apples. 40% is lost through cooking and is sensitive to light, air and alkaline conditions.

RDI: 1.0-2.2mg/day

Vitamin B12

Function: a co-enzyme in protein metabolism and has a key role in the synthesis of DNA and RNA. B12 is also found in bone marrow and nerve tissue where it participates in red blood cell production.

Deficiency: anaemia, lethargy, loss of appetite, lemon-yellow skin, weight loss and neurological disturbances, such as depression. The body has a very efficient method of storage and recycling of B12. Deficiency due to depletion takes 2—10 years to occur. B12 is sensitive to alkaline conditions but stable in heat, light, acid and oxygen.

Toxicity: is unlikely.

Food Sources: is produced by microbial synthesis, making mushroom/fungi and fermented food the best sources. Meat also contains high amounts.

RDI: 2µg/day

Vitamin C

Function: production and maintenance of collagen and connective tissue. Vitamin C is the body's antioxidant for the blood; it assists in wound healing, fights infections and slows down the degeneration of tissue. Vitamin C assists in iron absorption and is considered protective against cancer and heart disease.

Deficiency: scurvy (the degeneration of collagen, causing blood vessels to bleed, resulting in the destruction of biochemistry), bleeding gums, impaired wound healing. Vitamin C is easily destroyed during the cooking process, storage and pickling. There is also limited capacity for storage within the body.

Toxicity: rebound scurvy can occur when excessive and prolonged supplementation is suddenly ceased. There is also a risk of kidney stones, impaired cholesterol and folic acid metabolism; as well as interference with brain, nerve and thyroid function.

Food Sources: citrus fruits, berries, guava, paw paw, parsley, capsicum, cabbage, broccoli, Brussels sprouts and spinach.

RDI: 30-40mg/day

Vitamin D

Function: assists with calcium absorption for bone production and maintenance.

Deficiency: occurs when a person doesn't receive enough direct sunlight. Those at particular risk are infants, elderly people, those living in cold climates or wearing completely covered clothing for religious purposes. The result of deficiency is rickets (bendy bones), osteomalcia (impaired bone production) and osteoporosis (brittle bones).

Toxicity: no known effects.

Food Sources: is synthesised from sunlight by the skin. Food sources include butter, eggs and fish, but are considered insignificant. Supplementation is largely ineffective.

RDI: none set in Australia. USA has an RDA of 5μg/day

Vitamin E

Function: is an important antioxidant for the body. It works by protecting cell membranes and inhibiting LDL cholesterol oxidation. Vitamin E works with vitamin K in blood coagulation and is thought to be protective to the heart, eyes and spinal cord.

Deficiency: It is almost impossible to induce deficiency, but can occur in low birth weight, formula fed babies.

Toxicity: no known effects.

Food Sources: nuts, seeds, fish and most cooking oils. Almost all plant sources contain some vitamin E.

RDI: 7-10mg/day

Vitamin K

Function: mainly involved with blood clotting, but may also play a role in bone metabolism.

Deficiency: is extremely rare. Can cause blood haemorrhage and is routinely given to infants at birth.

Toxicity: can be potentially toxic if taken in large doses over a prolonged period of time.

Food Sources: spinach, soybeans, cabbage, green beans, oranges, apples and wheat bran. Vitamin K can be synthesised in the gut from intestinal bacteria, providing approximately 50% of the daily requirements.

RDI: 70-140µg

Calcium

Function: muscle contraction, nerve function, enzyme activity, blood clotting and bone formation.

Deficiency: many factors affect absorption including; vitamin D availability, sex hormones (oestrogen and testosterone are dependent on adequate fat intake), smoking, alcohol, salt intake, fibre and high protein diets, phytates and phosphate in milk. Sugar promotes absorption. Additionally, studies have shown that those who have a relatively low calcium intake will absorb higher amounts than those with a relatively high calcium intake. Calcium deficiency is mostly associated with osteoporosis, which commences in most people around the age of 30. This is when the epiphyses in the skeleton fuse and the laying down of bone density ceases. From this time onward the body is in maintenance mode, with the bones gradually becoming more brittle.

Toxicity: not heard of, as excess calcium is excreted in the urine, via the kidneys.

Food Sources: dairy, soft bone in canned fish, shellfish, nuts (particularly almonds and cashews), seeds (particularly sesame), parsley, figs and chives.

RDI: 800mg/day

Folate

Functions: crucial for DNA production, growth and repair of cells, red blood cell production and a healthy digestive tract. Very important during pregnancy.

Deficiency: spina bifida, neural tube defects and also associated with heart disease and cancer.

Toxicity: no known effects.

Food Sources: fortified cereals, nuts, chickpeas, avocado, oranges, spinach, broccoli, brussels sprouts, cabbage, peanuts, peas and wholemeal bread.

RDI: 200µg/day; 400µg/day during pregnancy

Iodine

Function: thyroid function, metabolic rate and the general growth and development of the central nervous system.

Deficiency: for the lifespan of a person, the requirement of iodine is about a teaspoon. Deficiency is common in places where soil levels are particularly low, such as Tasmania, India, Nepal, Indonesia, Papa New Guinea and the Philippines. Symptoms include goitre, cretinism and a low IQ.

Toxicity: is common in places like Japan where there is a high seaweed consumption, resulting in goitre and thyroid dysfunction.

Food Sources: found in plant and animal foods, however animal sources, except seafood, are considered not bio-available. Plant sources are 100% absorbed. These include: seaweed, fruits and vegetables, particularly root vegetables and those grown beneath the ground. Additional quantities occur in iodised table salt, food colourings and milk from cleaning product residue.

RDI: 0.2mg/day

Iron

Function: transportation of oxygen in the blood; release of energy from food; immune function and infection healing.

Deficiency: generally iron is efficiently recycled within the body. However, the demands of iron are the highest in children and women and when the dietary intake is inadequate anaemia can develop. Symptoms include: pale skin, orange coloured eye cavity, loss of appetite, shortness of breath and lethargy.

Toxicity: can be lethal, particularly with children who mistake iron supplements for lollies (candy). The body has no mechanism for excreting iron and is only lost through the loss of blood and the sloughing of the skin and gut.

Food Sources: is widely distributed in both plant and animal foods. However, animal sources (haem) are much easier for the body to absorb. Vegetarians really need to consume vitamin C rich foods with iron rich foods in order to maximize absorption. The best vegetarian sources include: dried fruit, lentils, legumes, chives, parsley, broccoli, spinach, nuts, and fortified breakfast cereals. Although breakfast cereals usually contribute about 40% of a person's iron intake (who consumes breakfast cereal), phytates from the husk inhibit iron absorption. This is compounded further by the consumption of tea or coffee.

RDI: 8-12mg/day

Magnesium

Function: bone formation, muscle contraction, nerve functions, protein synthesis and production of enzymes.

Deficiency: usually caused by alcoholism, over use of laxatives and bulimia. Symptoms include muscle weakness and heart arrhythmia.

Toxicity: no known effects.

Food Sources: present in most foods, but the best sources are cereals, grains, nuts and vegetables.

RDI: 300mg/day

Phosphorus

Function: works with calcium in bone and teeth formation. Also involved in the release and metabolism of energy.

Deficiency: very unlikely as is contained in all plant and animal food. However, phosphorus intake must not exceed that of calcium, as they must be consumed in the correct ratio. Otherwise, calcium will be purged from the body in order maintain the correct balance. Deficiency only occurs with starvation and eating disorders such as anorexia.

Toxicity: is unlikely, but will greatly impact calcium stores.

Food Sources: widely distributed in all plant and animal derived foods.

RDI: none set

Potassium

Function: one of the three major electrolytes in the body that controls fluid levels within the cells. Also has a vital role in muscle contraction, nerve impulses and the metabolism of carbohydrates and protein.

Deficiency: is unlikely.

Toxicity: when potassium is out of ratio with sodium it can cause elevated blood pressure leading to cardiac arrest.

Food Sources: widely distributed in all food.

RDI: 3000mg/day

Selenium

Function: important role in enzyme function.

Deficiency: only occurs in places where soil content is low. Symptoms include muscle weakness, inflammation and pain.

Toxicity: no effects known.

Food Sources: meat, fish, cereals, and root vegetables.

RDI: none set.

Sodium

Function: Vital for cell function and electrolyte mechanism.

Deficiency: very unlikely, as is generally over-consumed.

Toxicity: high sodium intake can cause high blood pressure, oedema (fluid retention), stroke, heart attack and stomach cancer. These health effects are caused when sodium and potassium cannot maintain their 1:1 ratio.

Food Sources: salt is abundant in most processed food and in small quantities in all unprocessed foods.

RDI: none set

Zinc

Function: carbohydrate metabolism, DNA synthesis, protein digestion, protein synthesis, bone metabolism, sperm production, growth and repair, would healing, immunity and sexual reproduction and development.

Deficiency: zinc intake is crucial in childhood and puberty to literally develop to one's potential. Symptoms include cracked or inflamed tongue and failure to thrive. Phytates in wholegrain cereals, tea and coffee can bind zinc making it bio-unavailable.

Toxicity: would only occur with supplementation and has been known to cause lethargy.

Food Sources: meat (muscle fibres), eggs, seafood, nuts, legumes, yeast and cereals.

RDI: 8mg/day

Phytochemicals and Flavonoids

Phytochemicals and flavonoids are little compounds that give plants their pigment and aroma. These compounds are mostly concerned with protecting the plant and keeping it healthy. A lot of research continues into phytochemicals and flavonoids in the belief that they can be just as beneficial to us. The consensus is that these wonderful substances have anti-cancer properties and may hold the key to curing many diseases. Flavonoids in particular seem to scavenge free radicals and have antimicrobial properties. Phytochemicals seem to be powerful antioxidants that have immuno-enhancement properties.

Obviously the health supplement industry couldn't wait to exploit the exciting prospects of these compounds. However, what has been found is there are various forms of each phytochemical and flavonoid and they seem to work synergistically, not individually. In addition, the bioavailability is uncertain when taken in supplement form. So as always, fresh is best!

An effective method of ingesting phytochemicals and flavonoids is by drinking freshly squeezed juice. The trick is to consume the juice within a maximum time period of twenty minutes from the moment the fruit or vegetable was cut. These compounds are very fragile, so the sooner they are consumed, the more likely they will be able to work their magic.

The phytochemicals are most commonly classified as the following, although more and more are being discovered.

Chlorophylls
Colour: green
Food Source: spinach, spring onions, green beans, peas, zucchini and leaves.
Part of Plant: leaves, stems and fruit.
Effect of Boiling: Unstable, up to 80% lost and generally insoluble in water.
Effect of pH: Lost in acidic conditions, prefers alkalinity.

Allicin
Colour: white
Food Source: garlic
Part of Plant: clove

Effect of Boiling: some loss in cooking

Effect of pH: not affected

Indoles

Colour: white, clear

Food Source: Asparagus, cauliflower, avocado, grapefruit, berries, brussels sprouts, broccoli, kale and onion.

Part of Plant: fruit flesh and pith

Effect of Boiling: many are activated during the cooking process. Can be soluble in water.

Effect of pH: not affected

Anthocyanins

Colour: yellow, red and purple

Food Source: onion, grapes, strawberries, cabbage and blueberries.

Part of Plant: flowers, roots and fruit

Effect of Boiling: stable with boiling but can be soluble in water.

Effect of pH: sensitive to pH changes.

Xanthophylls

Colour: green or yellow

Food Source: cabbage, broccoli, spinach, corn, paprika, zucchini, lettuce, cucumber, celery and leaves

Part of Plant: leaves, fruit and seeds

Effect of Boiling: not stable

Effect of pH: not affected

Carotenes

Colour: yellow, red or orange

Food source: carrots, tomatoes and capsicum

Part of Plant: leaves, stems and roots

Effect of Boiling: generally stable and soluble in water

Effect of pH: not affected

Flavonoids are as unique as the particular flavour of a fruit or vegetable and are therefore too many to mention.

The Super Foods

There are many foods that are touted as super foods and there are many lists available on the internet. My list has taken into consideration the amino acid profile as a complementary food; the vitamin and mineral content; or the presence of phytochemicals and antioxidant activity. While there are many more obscure foods that are attracting attention, I specifically decided to choose those that are readily available from the supermarket and won't break the bank.

Amaranth: An ancient grain that was used by the Inca people. It is often referred to as Inca wheat. Amaranth is a white lightweight grain that resembles tiny polystyrene balls. These balls have a perfect amino acid profile, making it a superior protein source. In addition, amaranth contains all minerals and most vitamins. There is virtually no taste and can easily be added to breakfast cereals, eaten as a porridge, used to replace breadcrumbs or made into delicious slices and biscuits (cookies).

Quinoa: Very similar to amaranth in its nutrient composition but denser in its vitamin and mineral content. The appearance of quinoa is of small creamy coloured hard balls. The flavour is quite nutty and can used as a rice or pasta substitute in risottos and stir-fries. It may also be eaten as porridge, made in to delicious salads or used in a variety of sweet delights.

Oats: This highly nutritious grain is a rich source of the B group vitamins, Vitamin E, K, folate and small amounts of most minerals. Oats are also high in fibre, particularly soluble fibre, giving them cholesterol-lowering properties and a low gylcaemic index. Oats are a particularly valuable food source for children and persons who are chronically ill or elderly.

Sunflower: An amazing plant that is entirely edible. The stems and flowers can be eaten raw or cooked. The seeds are delicious raw or roasted and the oil produced is highly nutritious. Throughout the plant, all vitamins and minerals are present. The seeds are high in zinc, iron, protein, calcium, thiamin, folate, phosphorus, niacin, mono-unsaturated fat and poly-unsaturated.

Garlic: These cloves are considered medicinal as they exhibit antibiotic and lipid lowering properties. Garlic has strong antioxidant and phytochemical activity. They have fair amounts of vitamin K, E, C, B1, B2 and most minerals. Garlic is mostly used as a flavouring agent in cooking, but is most potent when taken raw.

Parsley: A brilliant little herb that can be quietly slipped into salads, pastas, risottos and stir-fries. It is high in iron, calcium, folate, potassium, fibre, vitamin C and A. The flat leaf variety is a culinary delight and really easy to grow yourself.

Rocket: A great leaf that can be served raw or cooked. They are a rich source of vitamins and minerals, especially iron, calcium, folate vitamin A and C. Really easy to grow all year round.

Kale: Often called wild cabbage and is commonly used in soups and casseroles. It has high levels of phytochemicals, calcium, iron, folate, vitamin C, A, potassium, phosphorus and magnesium, also contains small amounts of zinc, tryptophan, sodium and niacin. Kale is easy to grow and can be added to many hot dishes to boost the nutrient density.

Soybeans: A fabulous little bean that is very popular in Asia. They are very high in protein, with most of the essential amino acids present. Soybeans are high in iron, folate, zinc, calcium, phosphate, potassium, niacin, magnesium, thiamin and most other vitamins and minerals. They also contain phytoestrogens, which are thought to be responsible for the low prevalence of breast cancer in China and Japan. Soybeans are available in many forms but are best consumed fresh straight from the pod.

Blueberries: These berries appear on most super food lists. They are well known for their potent antioxidant activity and are believed to have anti-cancer properties. Many cultures use blueberries to treat diarrhoea and stomach upsets. Blueberries are rich source of calcium, vitamin C, folate, magnesium, potassium, vitamin A and the phytochemicals carotene and anthocyanins. They are delicious fresh or made into sweet treats.

Figs: One of the most ancient of all crops, dating back 4,000 years. They are very high in most vitamins and minerals. Edible seeds like those found in figs are high in resistance starch, which are protective against bowel cancer. Figs are delicious fresh or dried.

Water

Water is the vital component of all living things, without it we die within a few short days. The average adult male has 60% water content, where as a woman has on average 51%. There is a potential to have as much as 80% water in the body, but unfortunately, most people do not drink enough water and are essentially dehydrated. Water provides the solution for chemicals to interact in the body. It also controls body temperature and eliminates waste products. Water is lost through the urine, bowel motion, sweating and breath.

Water must be replaced through food and drink, ideally two litres or 68floz from drinking water and an additional half a litre or 17floz contributed from the food intake. Just a 20% loss of water in the body will result in death. It always amazes me when people say they don't like water. I think you would be hard pressed to find an animal in nature that won't drink water because they 'don't like it'. The concept is ridiculous. So where did the sociably acceptable idea of sustaining oneself on tea coffee, cordial, juice and soft drinks come from?

Apart from herbal teas, none of the beverages mentioned above will actually quench the thirst. Since water is crucial to sustain life, why is it not the drink of choice and held in high regard? Next time you're refuelling your car, think how the engine would appreciate being run on coffee. The body really isn't any different and deserves a higher level of respect.

The urban rumour that when you feel the sensation of thirst, you are actually already dehydrated is true. The symptoms of dehydration include sunken features, particularly the eyes; dry loose skin, and in prolonged cases, kidney failure. Please endeavour to get your water quota each day. Carry a bottle and take small frequent sips.

Water composition varies according to its source. It would be foolish to think that water is just H2O. Only double distilled water is able to attain that kind of purity, tap water is somewhat different. A typical analysis of tap water varies in different locations, but usually contains: chlorine, monochloramine, trihalomethanes, aluminium, ammonia, calcium, chloride, chromium VI, copper, fluoride, iron, magnesium, nitrate, phosphorus, potassium, silica, sodium, sulphate and zinc.

It is unfortunate that fluoride has made its way in to most modern water supplies. We have falsely been informed that fluoride benefits us by reducing the prevalence of tooth decay. However, research shows that this simply isn't the case and that fluoride has absolutely no impact on dental health. In fact, fluoride is a highly toxic chemical which is a by-product of the fertiliser industry. Studies show that fluoride interferes with functioning of the central nervous system. In any other context it would be considered a hazardous pollutant, but when added to our drinking water it magically becomes a promoter of health.

Bottled water is typically labelled as 'natural spring' or 'mineral' water. Mineral water is purified water, usually by boiling with minerals dissolved. Typical composition includes: calcium, fluoride, chloride, sodium, magnesium and sulphate.

Natural spring water come from a natural undeground spring that is generally filtered through rocks. It receives no treatment other than filtration. Natural spring water is fairly stable in its composition but varies greatly according to location. A typical sample contains: calcium, sulphates, sodium, nitrates, chloride, manganese, magnesium, phosphate, potassium, and carbonates.

Natural spring water would be great if it wasn't for the plastic bottling. Polyethylene bottles, which are made from petro-chemicals, have been shown to allow its toxic chemicals to migrate into the water. On average bottled water contains 3.1% of various forms of benzene. Benzene is a highly toxic chemical and a known carcinogen. Bottled water is an unnecessary expense. I recommend carrying a stainless steel water bottle with you filled with filtered tap water. It is cheaper and healthier, just be wary of the cheap, plastic-lined stainless steel drink bottles. Filters generally remove chlorine, ammonia, lime, heavy metals, aluminium and residues from pesticides and fertilisers.

Phase Two—Those little unwanted extras in food

What are food additives and are they all bad?

The use of food additives was born straight out of the industrial revolution, where trickery and blatant highway robbery were the motivation. The use of food additives became more functional during the world wars, when scientists had a genuine need to prolong the lifespan of food. Today the use of food additives is widespread and a product often contains a cocktail of chemicals with unknown synergistic effects.

The *Food Standards Code*, describes a food additive as *"any substance not normally consumed as a food in itself and not normally used as an ingredient of food, but which is intentionally added to food to achieve one or more technological functions"*.

The avoidance of food additives must be a conscious decision, as they do seem to be in everything. All food additives are assigned an E number and unless you know what chemical the E number corresponds to, you may be left clueless.

Not all food additives are bad; some are vitamins, minerals and food acids, for example, citric acid. The trick is, knowing which processed foods have used the safer methods of preservation and which are potentially toxic. Of course the least amount of processing a food item has endured, the more likely it is to be healthy. However, the second phase doesn't need to be a Stone Age diet, there are plenty of foods on the market that have been processed with integrity.

At this stage, it doesn't mean never eating a favourite treat food again. You may find eventually, that the cravings for particular foods diminish and that you will start to view them differently. Let it take its natural course.

The function of food additives can be classified as follows:

Acidity regulator	Flavouring
Anti-caking agent	Flour treatment agent
Antioxidant	Glazing agent
Bulking agent	Intense sweetener
Bleaching agent	Humectant
Colour	Mineral salt
Enzyme	Preservative
Emulsifier	Propellant
Firming Agent	Stabilizer
Flavour enhancer	Thickener
Food acid	Vegetable gum
Foaming agent	

The main purpose of food additives today is profit making. Anyone who has worked in a supermarket will attest to the fact that stock turnover is very high. Bacon for example sells out all most daily and no one buys it with an intention to store it for lengthy periods. Salt and ascorbic acid (vitamin C) would be sufficient, otherwise why not sell it frozen? The bottom line is that additives are in use to satisfy global trade. Preservation is necessary, as the food will spend lengthy periods in shipping containers.

Buying local food reduces the food additive content and also sends the message to supermarkets that there is more market share in locally produced food.

The theory goes, that supermarkets stock shelves according to supply and demand. If a product doesn't sell, it is discontinued. Vote with your supermarket dollars for locally produced food, your own country is good, but your home state is even better.

Most foods could be preserved by the use of:

300	Vitamin C also known as ascorbic acid
306	Tocopherols also known as Vitamin E
307	γ-tocopherol
308	dl-α-tocopherol
309	δ-tocopherol

330   Citric acid
Freezing
Drying
Salting

The food additives to avoid and associated effects

Colours

Colouring agents are used purely for aesthetic purposes; they serve no other function other than looking good. There are three types of colours: naturally derived colours, like beetroot and paprika; chemically identical colours that are produced in a laboratory and are much cheaper than the natural counterpart; and the synthetic 'coal tar' colours, which are made from petro-chemicals. In Australia, there are thirteen coal tar colours still in use. It is important to note that natural colourings are still used in doses that exceed what they would in nature. 'Natural' colours or chemically identical colours are not consumed in 'natural' amounts and can still cause adverse reactions.

There are many colours that are shrouded in suspicion, however these are the colours where the evidence against their use is strong and have been banned elsewhere in the world. The Acceptable Daily Intake (ADI) in Australia is 290g/kg in food or 70mg/L.

102   Tartrazine
104   Quinoline Yellow
110   Sunset Yellow
122   Carmoisine
123   Amaranth
124   Ponceau 4R
127   Erythrosine
129   Allura red
132   Indigotine
133   Brilliant blue
142   Green S
153   Carbon Black

154	Brown HT
160b	Annatto extract*
174	Silver
175	Gold

All of these colouring agents are linked to hyperactivity, neurological disorders, migraines, skin rashes, asthma and eczema.

*Annatto extract has not been banned in other countries; however, double blind studies have shown it can cause hyperactivity (head-banging, oppositional defiance etc) and skin rashes in sensitive people. Annatto extract is used extensively through our food supply. The ADI varies with different food groups. The highest ADI for annatto extract is 100mg/kg in breakfast cereals. It is commonly found in cheese, butter, vegetable oil, ice-cream, yoghurt, biscuits, frozen chips and meat products.

Cochineal or carmines (120) are produced from beetles. It is the colouring that produces the pretty candy pink. It is used in pink icings, confectionary, ice-cream, cooking sauces, canned fruit, jelly, cakes, biscuits and marinades. The use of additive 120 is very widespread and is produced by boiling the beetles (sometimes just their wings) in acid and forming a concentrated powder. The powder is either used as is, or dissolved in alcohol and sold as 'natural' food colouring. I am certainly not against eating insects, most are highly nutritious; but I hardly see what is 'natural' about this process.

Sorbates

Sorbates are used to keep food moist, without mould forming. This type of preservative is linked to the trigger of asthma attacks and behavioural problems.

The highest ADI for sorbates is 1000mg/kg and are routinely used in the manufacture of confectionary, particularly fudge and ice confectionary. Other sources include cream cheese, dips, yoghurt, cheese rennet, sausages and fruit juice. It is possible to buy products without sorbates, always read the label.

| 200 | Sorbic acid |

201	Sodium sorbate
202	Potassium sorbate
203	Calcium sorbate

Benzoates

Benzoates are commonly used to prevent fruit products from fermenting or losing their flavour. Typical sources are soft drinks (soda), fruit juices, fruit tubs, fruit pies, yoghurt and cheese products. Benzoates form benzene when combined with vitamin C. Vitamin C is contained in most fruit or vegetable products. Benzene is a known carcinogen. Studies show that benzoates can cause hyperactivity, aggression, skin rashes and can trigger asthma attacks. The JENCFA database shows that test animals displayed hyper-excitability, incontinence, convulsions and all the animals died within two-weeks. Benzoates have an ADI of up to 2500mg/kg. Many products are free of benzoates, it is just a matter of reading the label.

210	Benzoic acid
211	Sodium benzoate
212	Potassium benzoate
213	Calcium benzoate

Propionates

Propionates are mould retardants; the most notable is 282, calcium propionate, which was famously exposed by Sue Dengate's double blind study. Results revealed that 282 could cause irritability, inattention; sleep disturbance, irritable bowel syndrome, heart palpitations, speech delay and lethargy. It was also found that the effects built up slowly and seem to accumulate in the body.

Propionates can be used at a level of up to 4000mg/kg and can be found in cakes, bread products and pastries. Many bakeries have removed the use of 282 in light of Sue Dengate's work, but commercial bread makers have become savvier. They use preserved vinegar and vegetable oil. When we were moving house I bought a loaf of commercial bread from the petrol station out of sheer desperation. For four days it sat on the bench and it was just as fresh as the day it was bought. Remember when buying a loaf of bread meant that it needed using up with in two days, beyond that it was toast or breadcrumbs. Breads containing vinegar were called sour dough. It is near impossible to find commercial bread that doesn't contain vinegar. In Australia, it is has been common practice to freeze bread as it has a tendency to get a little dry and chewy by the end of the day. I wonder if there is a need to do so anymore.

I recommend baking your own bread. If that isn't practical, go to a bakery and ask if there are preservatives added. The big bakery chains like Brumby's and Baker's Delight have stopped using propionates. However, I have discovered that they are still routinely used in rural locations. I think that is in a bakery's best interest not to use a preservative, as they bake fresh everyday. When the bread goes stale, you'll come back and buy more!

280	Propionic acid
281	Sodium propionate
282	Calcium propionate
283	Potassium propionate

Sulphites

Sulphites are mostly used to stop ingredients going brown or losing their colour. Mostly they are associated with asthma attacks. Research has shown that sulphite exposure irritates the airways, which exacerbates the effects of other known triggers. Sulphites are also linked to behavioural problems and stomach upset. JENCFA research indicated that doses between 250mg-6g caused vomiting and severe stomach and intestinal irritation in most of the human test subjects. In addition, sulphite intake caused increased calcium excretion, thiamin inactivation and the gradual depletion of vitamin A in the liver.

A small handful of dried fruit may contain 80mg of sulphite, yet the ADI is 0.7mg per kg of body weight. One sausage may contain 50mg. If you start adding up highly probable food sources that a small child might eat in any one-day, it greatly exceeds the

ADI. Sulphites are found in fruit juice, dried fruit, nuts, instant noodles, soup, muesli bars, breakfast cereal, fresh prawns, canned vegetables, cheese and wine, just to mention a few. Manufacturers can use sulphites up to a level of 3000 mg/kg depending of the type of food. It is possible to find food processed without the use of sulphites, it is just a matter of reading the label. It is even easier however, to choose fresh food over processed.

220	Sulphur dioxide
221	Sodium sulphite
222	Sodium bisulphite
223	Sodium metasulphite
224	Potassium metabisulphite
225	Potassium sulphite
228	Potassium bisulphite

Nitrates

Nitrates serve the function of a preservative but technically aren't classified as one and can legally be labelled as 'No Preservatives'. It is mostly used in fresh and cured meat products to prevent the growth of harmful micro-organisms. JENFCA strongly discourages the use of sodium nitrate in baby food or foods intended for small children. For this reason it is prohibited in baby foods. Unfortunately, sodium nitrate is used extensively in sausages, bacon, most crumbed or marinated meat, ham and other processed meats. Small children, even babies, commonly eat all of these foods. It would be appropriate to notify parents, so that they are able to make informed choices when feeding their children. Sodium nitrate consumption is associated with decreased growth, skin irritations, abdominal pain, headaches, nausea, confusion, dizziness and behavioural problems.

The nitrites are more toxic than the nitrates, but unfortunately nitrate can be converted to nitrite in the gut. Nitrate can also react with amines and form nitrosamine, which is a poison.

The highest ADI of nitrate or nitrite that can be used is 125mg/kg.

249	Potassium nitrite
250	Sodium nitrite
251	Sodium nitrate
252	Potassium nitrate

Antioxidants

Antioxidants sound healthy, but really aren't. These synthetic compounds prevent foods from going rancid from oxidation (exposure to oxygen and the micro-organisms that thrive in the presence of oxygen). They do not provide any health benefits. It has been found that 320 (BHA) and 321 (BHT) are readily absorbed in the fat tissue and takes three to four days to work its way through the system. This means that a regular consumption of foods containing BHA or BHT can result in an accumulation of the additives in the body, with higher levels than the recommended ADI. BHT was found in animal studies to elevate serum cholesterol. BHT was also found to interact with vitamin A to cause abnormalities in pregnancy and demonstrated a carcinogenic effect. BHT and BHA are prohibited for use in baby food or those intended for young children. It seems there is a need to inform pregnant women and parents of the dangers of BHT and BHA. Particularly, that these two additives often go undeclared in vegetable oil and commercial bread. These antioxidants are found wherever there is vegetable oil or animal fat and may be used at a level of up to 200mg/kg. The use of antioxidants can easily be avoided with the help of vitamin C, vitamin E, vacuum packaging, low temperature storage and storage away from light.

319	Tertiary butylated hydroquinone
320	Butylated hydroxyanisole
321	Butylated hydroxytoluene

Flavour Enhancers

Flavour enhancers particularly MSG are associated with 'Chinese Food Syndrome'. Due to the bad publicity, most Chinese food eateries proudly display a 'No MSG' sign. Of course this means that they're not sprinkling it into their dishes, but there have been several cases where ingredients have been used that already contain the flavour enhancer and have caused adverse reactions. Flavour enhancers are rarely labelled clearly and are often disguised as 'hydrolysed vegetable protein', 'yeast extract' or 'natural flavouring'. All are linked to headaches, insomnia, asthma, allergic reactions, hyperactivity and nausea.

627 and 631 are prohibited for use in baby food and 635 has been banned elsewhere in the world. In Australia, they are likely to be found in potato chips, sauces, marinades, sushi, burgers, fried chicken, spreads, instant noodles and frozen foods. There is no ADI set, which means that its use is unrestricted.

620	L-Glutamic acid
621	Monosodium L-glutamate (MSG)
622	Monopotassium L-glutamate
623	Glutamate
624	Monoammonium L-glutamate
625	Magnesium glutamate
627	Disodium 5'-guaylate
635	Disodium 5'-ribonucleotides
641	L-Leucine

Artificial Sweeteners

Artificial sweeteners are used to reduce the kilojoule or calorie content of food. Until recently, the evidence against artificial sweeteners was weak. The studies were poorly designed and not reasonably translatable to humans. Compelling evidence has emerged in recent years, resulting in serious doubts of the continued use of artificial sweeteners.

The research has focused on aspartame, which has been found can over stimulate the brain causing or exacerbating neurological disorders. In addition, animal studies show exposure to aspartame causes tumours. They also tend to have a laxative effect, which may interfere with nutrient absorption.

The current ADI varies according to its use, but the highest levels have been approved is for confectionary at a concentration of 10000mg/kg. Almost everything has a diet option that has been artificially sweetened.

951	Aspartame
952	Calcium cyclamate or sodium cyclamate
954	Saccharin
955	Sucralose
956	Alitame
957	Thaumatin
965	Maltitol
966	Lactitol
967	Xylitol

Carrageenan (407) is an emulsifier that is used in food to improve texture, as a thickening agent or to stop separation. It is currently allowed at a level of 2g/kg and often found in confectionary, dairy products, particularly ice-cream and infant formula. Studies on test animals show that carrageenan interferes with pepsin activity during the digestion process. This results in the interference of nutrient absorption, kidney damage and deformities.

Legally allowed residues in food

Most residues in food do not require labelling. Pesticides, nitrates from fertilisers, veterinary medications such as antibiotics and penicillin, hormones such as progesterone (only produced by females during pregnancy), cleaning fluids, insect particles, artificial ripening agents, radiation, saline solution (to add bulk to meat), processing chemicals such as sulphuric acid, caustic soda and hydrogen peroxide, and packaging migration, where chemicals from plastic, foil and ink make there way into processed foods and are legally considered perfectly acceptable in today's food supply.

The 5% labelling loophole and other labelling issues

In Australia, if an ingredient contained in a product is less than 5% of the overall formula it does not need to be labelled. This includes food additives. In addition, a product can claim to have 'no added preservatives' when the manufacturer has knowingly used an already preserved ingredient such as vegetable oil or vinegar. A common claim is 'No MSG' on a food label when another ingredient that is basically the same has been used. Hidden MSG sources include yeast extract, 627, 631, 635, hydrolysed vegetable protein and natural flavouring.

Hydrolysed vegetable protein is produced when scrap vegetables are boiled in a vat of sulphuric acid for several hours and then neutralised with caustic soda. The substance that is produced is dried and made into a powder. Ironically it can then be listed as a natural flavouring!

627 (sodium inosinate), 631 (sodium guanylate) and 635 (ribonucleotides) are the new breed of flavour enhancer and are up to 15 times stronger than MSG. As they are little known additives, the manufacturer can brazenly advertise the product as having 'No MSG'!

Another loophole that manufacturers exploit is the use of antioxidants. Antioxidants perform the same function as preservatives, but are technically not classified as one. Most people are under the illusion that antioxidants are good for us. The ones like vitamin C and Vitamin E are good for us, but the synthetic antioxidants like BHA and BHT are toxic.

Annatto extract (160b) is another additive that has been shown to cause adverse effects. It is often added to margarines, ice-creams, yoghurts, popcorn and biscuits to enhance the colour and flavour. As annatto is a plant extract it is often listed as 'natural flavouring' and on packets that say 'no artificial colourings or flavourings'.

Deception is rife in food labelling. It is interesting that section 3 volume 1 of the Codex Alimentarius (where most food legislation is derived) states *"no food should be in international trade which has in or upon it any substance in an amount which renders it poisonous, harmful or otherwise injurious to health.... it should not be labelled or presented in a manor that is false, misleading or deceptive".*

Many foods are now standardised, which means that the composition of ingredients cannot vary outside the guidelines. For example a product cannot claim to be meat based like a lasagne or a pie unless it contains at least 25% meat. Food additives can be compulsory in standardised foods unless the manufacturer can prove that the quality of the product is not compromised by their omission. This leaves the door open for food additives being used just for the sake of it.

Before The National Food Authority morphed into Food Standards Australia and New Zealand (FSANZ), an additive could only be approved if it could establish that a satisfactory product could not be manufactured without the requirement of the particular food additive. We now have a system where the manufacturer, not our regulating body FSANZ, carries out biochemical safety tests. The testing is performed on animals such as mice, rats, dogs, monkeys, hamsters, rabbits and cattle—very rarely on humans. Cellular and DNA testing is performed. Behaviour and psychological effects are not considered in the outcome.

A test animal is fed quantities of a food additive until any adverse effects are observed. Inter-reactions with other food additives are not considered. The NOEL (No Observed Effect Level) is used to create an ADI (Acceptable Daily Intake). The ADI is set at 1/100 of the maximum NOEL of the most sensitive test animal. A chemical's safety is dependant on the assumption that a human is 10 times more sensitive than a test animal. The problem with that is sometimes humans are more sensitive than the test animals. BHT and BHA were found to accumulate in the adipose tissue (fat store) at higher levels than the test animals used to approve to chemical in 1965.

The World Health Organisation (WHO) and The Joint Expert Committee of Food Additives (JECFA) develop the principles for the evaluation of foods additives. The outcomes of these evaluations are generally adopted in Australia without further independent testing. In other words if a manufacturer wants to use an additive and JECFA has deemed it safe, it will generally be approved. Other countries' regulating bodies perform their own safety tests before approval of food additives. As that step is skipped in Australia, there are numerous food additives that are permitted for use that have been banned elsewhere in the world. These include: 102, 104, 110, 120, 122, 123, 124, 127, 129, 132, 133, 142, 151, 153, 155, 173, 174, 175, 320, 285, 635, 952 and 954.

As it turns out many of the food additives used today were approved during the period of 1965 to 1966. Even when there is irrefutable evidence, like the effects of tartrazine, legislation has a habit of being stubborn, particularly when there are manufacturers eager to continue its use. Some countries, particularly Norway has set their own standards. While Australia has 877 colouring agents approved for commercial use, Norway has just 34.

The United Kingdom recently banned the use of coal tar colours following government funded and university studies revealed adverse reactions. In addition, the United Kingdom has also moved to ban the combination of benzoates and vitamin C, such as in fruit juice, as the combination was found to form benzene, a known carcinogen. As a result, manufacturers including Nestle and Cadbury have changed their recipes to now exclude the use of coal tar colourings. It is interesting those same companies are still using their original formulas in the products intended for other countries, including Australia.

There are about 1000 food additives that have been approved for use in Australia; this number has more than doubled in the past twenty years. This figure doesn't include the several thousand 'flavours' that are approved for use without labelling requirements.

There are some labelling laws that are fairly well regulated. These are nutrient claims such as 'low fat' or 'reduced fat'. In order for a product to be labelled as 'low fat', it must not contain more than 3g fat per 100g or 3% fat in the overall product. 'Reduced fat' is when a product has been reduced in fat content by 25% of the original formula. 'Fat free' must not contain more than 0.15g fat per 100g. A product labelled 'low in sugar' must not contain more than 3g of sugar per 100g or 3% sugar in the overall product. Sugar is often labelled as carbohydrates, and it can be difficult to differentiate between added sugar and those derived from complex carbohydrates such as flour, wholegrains or fruit.

Of course the food industry always finds a way to side step around legislation. And so the terms 'light' and 'lite were born. Legally the label must specify in what way the product is light/ lite. However this type of claim has become a clever way to market a product when it doesn't satisfy the criteria of the 'low' or 'reduced' classifications.

Ultimately, if the consumer wants to know exactly what is contained within a product, a phone call to the manufacturer is required. As multinational corporations control the bulk of our food supply, consumer hotlines are usually printed on a label.

Preservation Techniques

The purpose of preservation is to deter the growth of micro-organisms, which can cause food-borne illness such as salmonella. Food generally needs to be stored below 5°C or above 60°C to destroy the conditions necessary for micro-organisms to thrive. This is why you should never accept warm sushi or a cold burger.

Preservation of food has been part of culture for thousands of years, through the use of drying, salting and pickling. In the last hundred years it has become progressively more sophisticated. Most people would be familiar with canning, freezing, blanching and possibly Ultra High Temperature (UHT) where products like milk are subjected to high heat for a few seconds. In recent years food technology has taken giant leaps. Preservation techniques such as irradiation, high-pressure treatment, micronisation, super-critical extraction, active packaging, modified atmosphere, microwaving and pasteurisation are now common place.

Freezing is definitely the best method of preservation. Fruits, vegetables, meat and left over meals can be stored at

-18°C for three to twelve months with minimal nutrient loss. With the exception of meat, freezing will damage the cell membrane making cooked or blanched foods better suited to freezing than fresh foods. Commercial vegetable companies usually snap freeze their produce shortly after harvest and are therefore subjected to fewer preservation techniques.

Blanching and UHT treatment will result in a 10-20% loss of most vitamins and minerals.

The method of canning results in a loss of up to 50% of carotenes; an 80% loss of vitamin C; a 60% loss of B group vitamins; a 100% loss of riboflavin and a 70% loss of thiamin. Canned foods are high in amines and are susceptible to the food-borne illness, botulism.

Pasteurisation is a term that most people are familiar with; it is used extensively with dairy products and fruit juice. It is uses one of two heating methods: 80°C for 5 seconds or 65°C for 30 minutes. Nutrient losses are between 10-25%. It is interesting to note, that if a calf were fed pasteurised, homogenized milk, it would soon die.

Irradiation

Involves the use of X-rays, beta rays and gamma rays. Different levels of radiation are used for a variety of desired effects, such as to delay maturation of fruit, inhibit sprouting and destroy pathogens, bacteria and parasites. Radiation is very harmful to all living things with the exception of viruses and bacterial toxins, which can be very resistant to radiation.

Onions, potatoes and garlic are routinely irradiated to inhibit sprouting. The acceptable level is 0.1-3kGy. Fruits, grains and flour are irradiated to control insects, with an acceptable level of 0.2-0.7kGy. All meat is approved for irradiation, but pork is treated routinely to kill parasites such as, Toxoplasma gondii, Trichinella and Opisthorchis, at a dose of <1kGy. Frozen poultry, seafood and spices are given the largest dose of 3-10kGy to destroy salmonella, e coli, Listeria, campylobacter and shillelagh. Fruits, particularly those intended for export are treated with a dose of 2-5kGy in order to delay maturation.

Irradiation was initially introduced in 1989 in Australia as a three-year government trial to determine its safety. The trial was then extended under the guise of developing a national standard. In the meantime, the WHO and The International Atomic Energy Authority approved the use of irradiation and it was used unregulated in Australia until 1995. Australia then developed its own guidelines and restricted the use of irradiation to tropical fruit, herbal teas and spices. Tropical fruit and herbal teas may receive a dose of 10kGy and spices may receive 30kGy. Foods that have been treated must be labelled.

Irradiation is now used extensively throughout the world with an acceptable level of up to 50kGy in use. It is still unclear how much radiation is retained within the food, but as radiation damages cellular DNA and we are then ingesting the radiation, it is of concern. Food Standards Australia and New Zealand maintain its use is safe, but won't comment on why irradiation was restricted to a few items. As much of our food supply is imported, it begs the question, "How well is the imported irradiated food regulated?" I'm yet to see a sign up in front of any tropical fruit stand that declares the use of irradiation, that the food standards code states is mandatory.

High Pressure Treatment

Involves the use of electrical impulses of 10-20kV/cm. This method is predominately used on fruits and vegetables and works by rupturing the cell membrane. As a result, the life force of the produce is liberated; rendering it dead before it even reaches the supermarket shelf.

Microwave

This method is used to kill micro-organisms by thermal effect. It only works in products where there is sufficient contained water to allow the agitation of the molecules.

Micronisation

Infrared is used to destroy micro-organisms and enzymes in fruits and vegetables. It is also used to thicken liquids such as soup. A wavelength of 1.8-3.4μm is used for approximately five minutes.

Super critical extraction

Commonly uses carbon dioxide at a temperature of 31.1°C to extract a variety of substances from whole foods. This method is used to extract substances like vitamins and oils to make health supplements. It is also used to decaffeinate coffee and make various spice extracts. It is also the basis of reducing fat or cholesterol content in food in order to make the low fat varieties.

Active packaging and Modified atmosphere

A novel way to extend the shelf life of food and often is used in tandem to preserve highly perishable items like yoghurt or cottage cheese. It uses gases such as nitrogen and carbon dioxide to reduce oxygen levels. In other words the space between the edible portion and the lid is filled with a gas to displace the area that would ordinarily be occupied by oxygen. Many micro-organisms are aerobic, which means they are oxygen dependant. Removing the oxygen reduces the risk of food-borne illness. The active packaging component is usually on the foil lid or on the synthetic lining of a steel or plastic lid. The lid is impregnated with oxygen scavengers. So it might be time to rethink licking the foil lid!

The lengths we go to in order to have a life of convenience seems absurd. The reality is that food decomposes and once micro-organisms start to thrive, food becomes potentially lethal. Plying our food with chemicals just doesn't make sense. Wouldn't it be more logical to eat our food fresh the way nature intended?

Naturally occurring toxins in food

The food we eat today has literally come about by trial and error. The truth is that many naturally occurring plants are toxic, even lethal. The crops that have developed are mainly because of three factors: flavour, economics and not making the masses sick.

Would it surprise you to know that cabbage contains arsenic or that there is enough cyanide in a cup of apple seeds to kill a person?

The following is a list of naturally occurring toxins and the associated effects.

Mercury: Levels are steadily increasing due to mining pollution and natural erosion. The highest concentrations occur in the largest fish of the food chain, such as tuna, salmon, swordfish, halibut, shark and shellfish. Smaller fish such as herring, bream, whiting and sardines have relevantly low levels of mercury. Fish that is likely to be caught off a beach or jetty is likely to contain a tiny amount of mercury, where as those caught in deep-sea fishing are likely to have significant amounts. The Maximum Tolerable Amount (MTA) is 5µg per kg of body weight per week. The problem with mercury is that only small amounts can be excreted by the body and therefore accumulates over time. Majority of the mercury accumulates in the kidneys, liver and brain.

Mercury has been found to cause acute poisoning, kidney damage, sensory nerve damage, hearing defects and visual disturbances. In severe cases of poisoning, death will occur.

Mercury exposure during pregnancy is highly correlated with the incidence of cerebral palsy and retardation. An intake of 0.3mg per day over a prolonged period of time would normally result in poisoning.

Canned tuna contains approximately 0.32mg/kg of mercury. Canned salmon generally isn't an issue as most salmon is farmed instead of wild.

Glycoalkaloids: Found in potatoes and known as 'potato poisoning'. They reach harmful levels when potatoes are exposed to light, causing the greening effect. The greening is actually chlorophyll forming, which allows glucoalkaloids to thrive. Potatoes that have started to sprout can be up to 17 times higher in glucoalkaloid concentration. But some potatoes without greening or sprouting can contain harmful levels. It is always wise to peel potatoes and discard the skin. Symptoms of potato poisoning include nausea, headaches, vomiting, mental confusion, depression and drowsiness.

Cadmium: Found in most plant food and omnivorous animals. Cadmium is a non-essential metal that is absorbed from the soil and occurs alongside zinc. Cadmium can leach from cooking utensils, enamel cookware and pottery glazes.

Exposure seems to have an effect on calcium absorption and is also linked to prostate cancer. Cadmium does not cross the placenta, so starts to accumulate after birth, mostly in the liver and kidneys. While up to 90% is excreted, the residual is stored for an estimated 18 years.

The MTA is 7μg per kg of body weight. Levels of 0.5mg per 100g can be found in chocolate and peanuts. Vegetables, rice and wheat generally have 0.1mg per 100g of cadmium.

Lead: The neurological and poisoning effects of lead is well known, particularly in paint. Lead can be found in drinking water, seafood, plant and animal derived food. The MTA is 5μg per kg of body weight per week. Fish may contain 0.5mg/kg; lambs' liver may contain 0.35mg/kg; cereal grains may contain 0.2mg/kg and fruit and vegetables my contain 0.1mg/kg.

Arsenic: A known poison is contained in seafood, cereal and the humble cabbage. Symptoms include vomiting, diarrhoea, thirst and weakness.

Hydrogen cyanide: Highly toxic, can be lethal. Found in small quantities in cassava, lima beans, apricot kernels, almonds and apple seeds.

Glucosinolates: Can cause goitres if consumed in large quantities. Found in brussels sprouts, cabbage, cauliflower, turnip and mustard.

Nitrates/Nitrites: Has the same effects as the food additive varieties. Found in low levels in cabbage, celery, lettuce and spinach.

Oxaltes: Associated with decreased calcium absorption. Found in rhubarb, spinach and tea.

Psotalens: Found to be carcinogenic and a mutagen. Found in celery and parsnip.

Caffeine: May seem harmless, but is a drug that is widely over-consumed. The effects of caffeine are individual and dose related, some of which include: cardiac stimulation; increased gastric secretion and may relax the smooth muscle. Try giving it up and you'll see what a powerful drug it actually is.

Going Additive Free

A chemical elimination diet can be a very sobering experience. Many people I have interacted with will tell me that they don't believe that food additives affect them. So did I. When I underwent a three-week chemical elimination diet out of support for my then eight-year-old daughter. I was truly startled. Initially I experienced what I can only describe as withdrawal symptoms. The first week I was very snappy and easily irritated. Of course it didn't help that I had a daughter who was displaying similar symptoms. By week two, I felt that I was sleeping much better and was waking up feeling remarkably bright and fresh. At that time *'Brain Training'* on *Nintendo DS* and *'The Big Brain Academy'* on *Nintendo Wii* were popular in my house (and in general!). I recorded my lowest 'brain age' of twenty-two and both my daughter and I were performing much better than usual on *'The Big Brain Academy'*. Overall, I felt more alert, calmer, patient and people didn't seem to irritate me as much, particularly on the road, or waiting in queues. I had to admit, that I was very apparently affected by food chemicals.

My eldest daughter had undergone extensive medical testing after she was diagnosed with juvenile bipolar disorder. I had seen on a talk show that true bipolar would show up on an EEG test (brain scan). Instead of taking the prescription for mood altering drugs that my daughter's paediatrician was insisting was necessary, I asked for a referral to a neurologist. The EEG and CAT scan proved that there was nothing inherently wrong with her brain, it even ruled out ADHD, which can also be diagnosed with an EEG. When I returned to the paediatrician, he suggested a chemical elimination diet to see if food was an issue. Interestingly, the prescription for mood stabilisers was still on offer.

The chemical elimination diet was a conscious commitment at first. As I was already a qualified nutritionist our diet was already fairly healthy, but it was high in salicylates (found in fruits and vegetables), amines (found in cheese, fruits and vegetables), benzoates (found in yoghurt, juice boxes and fruit tubs), annatto extract (found in muesli bars, yoghurt, microwave popcorn, ice-cream and commercial biscuits) and calcium propionate (found in bread, cakes, pastry and pizza bases) Our seemingly healthy diet was actually quite high in reactive food chemicals.

My daughter had always suffered from extreme eczema. Over the years I had literally tried every cream and wives tales known to man. Different remedies helped, but nothing cured her condition. Her skin felt like sandpaper and her feet were like split tomatoes. Everyday I used to steri-strip her wounds together just so she could walk. After two weeks on the chemical elimination diet, my daughter's eczema literally disappeared; her skin was remarkably baby-smooth. In addition, the wild look in her eyes disappeared along with her highly erratic, unreasonable behaviour.

I realised that she had been intoxicated all these years and trying to reason with her was like trying to reason with a person high on drugs or alcohol. Three years later life is much different. She's still a kid and gets into trouble, but I can reason with her now, when before it was like talking to a brick wall. When my daughter comes into contact with foods she will react to, like at a birthday party, her lips will crack and bleed, she'll get red streaky lines down her face and she tells me that she feels different. The school reports that come home now make me so proud. It is so nice so have put an end to the constant meetings with her teachers, deputy principals, school psychologists, and the scathing school reports I used to receive.

I recommend a three-week chemical elimination diet by avoiding the worst of the food additives (coal tar colours, benzoates, nitrates, sulphites, propionates, artificial sweeteners and BHT/BHA) and following a low to moderate salicylate and amine diet. This can easily be achieved by consuming fresh food and only small amounts of processed food.

At the end of the three-weeks, introduce one type of additive at a time. In the first week, try some coloured foods. Wait at least three days and try benzoates. Work your way through the different food additives and observe any change in behaviour or skin appearance. The effects are usually quite obvious and individual tolerance levels vary. Some people are also affected by salicylates and amines, which will be discussed further in the next chapter.

Phase Three—Go Organic

What does it mean to eat organically?

The term 'organic' can be quite dubious, as everything is organic is someway. To be certified organic, it means that the product must be produced without the use of any pesticides, fungicides or synthetic fertilisers. It does not guarantee that ripening has taken place naturally or it has escaped cold storage. The regulation is not uniform throughout the world, although currently there is an international 'gold standard' being developed.

Changes in agricultural methods and hybridisation of fruit and vegetables have resulted in a dramatic fall in nutrient levels. Prior to World War II agricultural chemicals were virtually unused. By 1995, more than forty-five million tonnes of chemical fertilisers were used in the US alone. Now 95% of the world's crops are produced with chemical fertilisers and pesticides.

Research indicates that fruit and vegetables produced by traditional organic methods have superior protein and amino acid profiles. In addition there is on average 19% more iron, 22% more calcium, 43% more sodium, 14% more potassium, 81% more copper, 37% magnesium and up to 50% more vitamins, particularly vitamin C. Fourteen separate studies have all found similar results.

Pesticides, insecticides, weedicides, antibiotics and hormones are routinely used in agriculture to keep plant and animal yields high. There are over a hundred chemicals that are approved for use and they are almost always used in tandem with something else. For example, an apple tree will usually have the full spectrum of allowable chemicals used, wheat will have approximately eighty different chemicals applied during its growing season and broccoli will receive about sixty-five.

The toxicity and level of residue retained by each pesticide varies. Wholemeal bread may contain 0.59mg/kg of pesticide residue; bran may contain 1.78mg/kg and human milk (yes, it passes through the breast milk to our babies) contains on average 0.06mg/kg.

The pesticides and their residues are known or suspected carcinogens. Fortunately, the very worst pesticides have been banned. Up until about twenty years ago, hydrogen benzenes were used. These compounds contained benzene rings, which are the most stable form of compound known to science. It is estimated that the contaminated soil would take fifty years (if ever) to break down these highly toxic pesticides.

Eating organically doesn't necessarily mean spending a fortune on certified organic produce. Most of us are capable of growing a few veggies at home. Obviously, I am not suggesting that everything must be home-grown as climates differ, as does available space. However, most people I am sure have the ability to grow salad and other basic vegetables. Fruit can be more challenging, as fruit trees can occupy a lot of space and don't fair as well in pots. We devote so much space to having a front lawn. I recently visited Nepal and noticed that every front yard was growing a variety of vegetables, grain and fruit. Even the hotel I stayed in was completely self-sufficient. What is so aesthetically pleasing about a front lawn? So many of us spend a lot of money and effort into having the perfect lawn. Perhaps the Nepalese have the right idea and it is time to rethink this concept.

Not all of us live in the suburbs with a surplus of space; plenty of people live in apartment complexes. In that case, I recommend the use of hanging baskets, windowsills and compact planter boxes. Hopefully, there is an organic farmer's market within reasonable vicinity as they are worth the travel. If you are fortunate to live near an old-fashioned allotment, rent a patch!

The bottom line is that food was not intended to be produced with a host of chemicals and under Frankenstein conditions. Fruit and vegetables should be allowed to ripen naturally and eaten in a timely fashion. Animals intended for food should have space to move and fed a diet that is close to their natural diet. Accelerated growth hormones, antibiotics, artificial ripening and genetic modification, is just not what nature intended. It comes back to the market share concept; when people accept inferior food, it will continue to be produced. Our shopping dollars count.

I certainly appreciate what it is like to be on a budget. It's really tough to consider the world when it's a battle just to put food on the table. There was once a time when I had only fifty dollars left over after rent and bills to buy food and put petrol in the car. I ate eggs from my grandparents' chickens—a lot! I learnt that cooking from scratch is much cheaper than buying pre-packaged food. I learnt to be creative. There is time involved, but imagine what it was like for women fifty plus years ago before the days of washing machines, dishwashers and microwaves. With the help of machinery, I can make many things from scratch, with very little effort. Over the past decade, food has become very expensive. When I buy convenience foods, my weekly grocery bill is approximately four hundred dollars. When I make my own and grow my own my family consisting of four children can be fed on about one hundred and fifty dollars per week. To buy organic bread, pasta, yoghurt and biscuits etc would be very costly. Instead, buy organic flour, milk and eggs and there won't be much that can't be made from scratch at a fraction of the price. Before you say "I don't have time!" Start assessing how much time you spend watching television or at the computer, it adds up surprisingly quick! My life is made possible, as I only watch one or two movies per week, and spend about an hour on the internet each night. It can be done. Start wondering if you really came to Earth to check out what's on TV and I guarantee, you'll find an extra five hours each week very easily.

Phase three is actually more about becoming conscious, taking our place in nature, losing the shackles of society constraints and realising what is really of value in life. When we start to appreciate ourselves as creatures of earth instead of citizens and consumers, life becomes a lot less complicated.

Meat Production

Gone are the days when the bulk of the meat supply was produced with integrity. Trickery with food dyes and saline solution has been around for centuries, but at least the meat came from animals that had the liberty of pastureland and a natural diet. In Australia, about 40% of our meat supply and 80% of meat from large supermarkets come from feedlot operations. Animals are confined in pens and are fed by unnatural means. Animals that aren't able to move adequately have weaker muscles and a poor amino acid profile. Therefore confined animals produce low quality meat. Research shows that iron and zinc levels have fallen approximately 50% over the past fifty years.

Chicken Production

In Australia, the average person consumes 35kg of chicken per year. Most of us would rarely give a thought as to how that chicken was raised. Unless it is advertised as 'free-range' it was most likely raised in a 150m x 15m shed. Each shed contains up to 50,000 chickens. The floor consists of a litter that could be sawdust, rice hulls or rammed earth. At best the litter is changed after the batch of chickens are removed for slaughter. However, multi-batching or partial cleaning is perfectly acceptable.

The air quality is poor and they are known for catching six types of illness, including two types of respiratory disease. As the regulators are more concerned with the outside air pollution, the chickens are subjected to a slow-flow air ventilation system.

The chickens are kept without natural sunlight, some are given artificial lighting during the daytime until the time they are rounded up in the dead of night, usually between five and eight weeks old and taken off for slaughter.

The legislation is mostly focused on noise, dust and odour emissions; there is little concern for animal welfare.

Egg Production

The battery egg industry is notoriously unsavoury. Chickens are kept confined in cages; their feet often grow to be fused to the wire cage. They are basically biological machines. The chickens are fed a cocktail of antibiotics and hormones, as well as being fed a diet that is far from natural. By the time the chickens are excused from their laying duties, they are barely able to walk and have lost most of their feathers. The end of the road for these battery hens is being slaughtered for pet food, often dropped directly into a grinder while still alive.

Organic free-range eggs come from chickens that can move around freely in outdoor areas. They generally do not roam 'free', but at least the chickens can scratch in the dirt, flap their wings and experience fresh air and sunlight. The diet the chickens have is organic, natural and free of veterinary medications and hormones.

Beef Production

Feedlots in Australia were non-existent until 1994, until the Federal government heavily promoted the establishment of a feedlot industry. It's hard not to wonder why in a country that is so vast why exactly this was necessary. Apparently our beef wasn't cheap enough, we needed to stay competitive in the export market and supply supermarkets with 80% of their discount beef. There are various classes of feedlot operations, some are better than others, but as the set up cost is high, the feedlot tends to be run like a factory.

The feedlots range in size between 9m² to 25m², with the larger size holding up to 1000 head of cattle. The floor is generally concrete, but is sometimes rammed earth or metal grills. Many of the operations are based on once or twice per day feeding systems and are mostly comprised of corn. This is an animal that would ordinarily graze continuously on grass. Corn makes the cow rapidly gain weight and is not exactly the natural diet of a cow. In addition, each cow gets a 3cm or 1.2 inches allowance at the water trough, which is barely enough room to get a drink.

Occasionally the cows are provided shade, but it is not a requirement. In South Australia they decided that the National Guidelines were not stringent enough and needed more detail.

Subsequently, the South Australian guidelines ask those applying for a license to factor in the climate for the proposed feedlot and suggest a minimum of 2.5m² per animal. The legislation is still mostly concerned with human and environmental impact.

My research found that the smaller the slaughterhouse, the more likely the cows are treated with respect. The larger processing plants are automated factories, which can be inhumane and down right cruel. Organic farming doesn't necessarily guarantee a kinder slaughtering method. However, the likelihood of ethical animal treatment increases in the organic, free-range farming industry.

Pork Production

Feedlot piggeries have been in use for a very long time. Some are group penned, some are in individual stalls and others are in deep litter houses, a bit like the chickens. The pigs raised in group stalls have an allowance of 1m². The individually penned pigs have an area of 0.6m x 2.2m, which does not allow the pig to turn around, they can move back and forward slightly. The deep litter houses are probably the best scenarios. The pigs are housed together on a sawdust or similar flooring. A sow will have 1.5m²; a boar will have 2m² and a lactating sow with piglets will have 6m². Most of them will never see the light of day. You can tell the pigs that have never seen sunlight, as their skin is very pale and soft. Free-range pigs get quite a tough, darker skin that makes great crackling!

A free-range piggery, chicken or cattle farm is much cheaper to set up and has lower running costs. The animals are happier, the meat is of a superior quality and we are not short of space in Australia—it's a no-brainer really. The feedlot system is driven by greed. The average farmer isn't using this system, in fact there are only about seven hundred feedlots operating in Australia. Where I live, farms with cows and sheep surround me. They are real families that are battling to make a living. Smaller farmers are being undercut by the feedlot operators (which are very expensive to set up) and have now taken 40% of the market share. I believe that it is worth paying a few dollars more per kilo or pound at the butcher and support the farmers who are doing the right thing.

Tricks of the trade

The use of hormones to help animals grow faster was exposed a few years ago. However, unless the meat is labelled as 'hormone free', assume that it isn't. The hormone most commonly used is progesterone, a pregnancy hormone. It makes animals grow much faster than usual and much bigger than is naturally possible. This means that animals can be slaughtered sooner, feed expenses are reduced and overall the profit margin is increased. Residue of the progesterone can be found in the meat and there has been a lot of speculation of what possible consequences there could be for the male population and the pre-pubescent female population.

Antibiotics are routinely used to treat or prevent illness in the stock animals. Residues of the antibiotics are found in meat and also dairy produce. Dairy cows are routinely treated for mastitis. It has been widely reported that the over use of antibiotics has led to the development of super-bugs.

Saline solution is used to plump up the meat so that the weight is exaggerated, resulting in a greater profit margin.

Selecting organic animal products

Selling perishable items is a risky business, so it's understandable that proprietors would go to considerable lengths to prolong the saleability of their products. Breadcrumbs, marinades and food colourings are used to disguise the appearance, texture and odour of 'older' meat. Sodium and potassium nitrate/nitrite, as well as sulphur dioxide are used to delay rancidity. Fresh meat is frozen and thawed out again the next day and sold as fresh. The more worrying occurrence is the use of vacuum packaging. Meat sold in vacuum packaging is often up to ten weeks old. Vacuum sealing eliminates oxygen and therefore prevents bacteria from growing. However, amines don't need oxygen to thrive. Amines are compounds that are inevitable in the presence of cellular death—they are the result of decay or protein denature (oxygen causes the foul odour). The slimy substance on vacuum packed meats and bacon or ham is amines. Canning is similar to vacuum sealing where amines still thrive.

Amines

Amines are derivatives from ammonia. Not all are bad; in fact many such as amino acids are vital for bodily function. However, some amines can accumulate in the body causing toxic effects, such as headaches, tiredness, irritability, inattention and a lack of motivation and focus. Everyone's tolerance for amines is different, but the end result is intoxication. Hay fever is an example of how some people react to histamines.

The boiling point of amines are very high and therefore heat stable during normal cooking. Amines are commonly found in meat, fish, cheese and some over-ripe fruit and vegetables, particularly tomatoes, plums and grapes.

Some people can be severely affected by amines and need to avoid them altogether. Many people who suffer from depression or migraines can really benefit from eliminating amines from their diet. The effect of amines can be assessed in the same manner as food additives with a chemical elimination diet. The elimination should focus heavily on not consuming cheese, wine, meat, fish, tomatoes and grapes for at least two weeks.

Be an informed consumer

It is reasonable to ask your local butcher when an animal was slaughtered, if they use preservatives and if they purchase meat from feedlot producers. A good butcher will happily disclose this information. A dodgy butcher, who is trying to make money at your health's expense, will be evasive.

Organic free-range meat is obviously the way to go, but the mark up can be considerable. My honest opinion is that it is better to eat meat less frequently, that is of a high quality, than to eat inferior meat frequently. The Mediterranean diet, which is regarded by nutritionists as one of the most healthy ways to eat, is based on the consumption of red meat one-two times per month. There is so much status tied up with eating red meat, it is just over-spill from The Great Depression and the World Wars. Given that health professionals recommend meat consumption a maximum of three times per week, maybe its time to change our mindset about vegetarian food.

Salami and sausages really should be avoided. They are not actually classified as meats due to the lack of meat content. There are also links to cancer, not to mention a complete lack of nutrients. I understand that everyone loves a snag at a barbecue and that's fine. Like I have stated, the body is very resilient. It is the weekly consumption as a family staple that is of concern.

Food dye is often added to give cuts of meat that bright red appearance. It is really unnatural for meat to look that way so why do consumers find it so appealing?

Fresh cuts are never used in marinated or crumbed varieties, so always buy the meat fresh and marinate or crumb it yourself.

If you accept substandard food, expect that the farmer, butcher and supermarket will keep supplying it. Cut back on meat consumption and make a commitment to only buy meat that has been produced with integrity, even if it is more expensive. When the demand for fresh organic free-range meat increases, the supply will increase and therefore the price will decrease. It's economics, not rocket science.

Cold storage and artificial ripening

Many of us would have no idea how most fruits and vegetables actually taste. This is because fruits and vegetables are routinely picked before the ripening stage is complete. The produce is placed into a cold storage facility and then artificially ripened when required. There are many consequences of this practice.

Firstly, the fruit or vegetable is denied of maturing naturally, which prevents the natural flavour from developing. This also means that the nutrient composition fails to reach is maximum potential.

The cold storage facilities are very costly operations. Initially all produce is washed with chlorine and then place in large sheds that work by modifying the atmosphere. This usually involves pumping carbon dioxide into the room to reduce the oxygen levels and therefore decreasing the microbial activity. Other systems are based on the use of antibiotics and propylene glycol. The antibiotics prevent bacteria and mould forming; where as the propylene glycol assists with moisture retention.

While short periods of cold storage have shown to cause very little damage to nutrient content and quality, long-term storage has shown a deterioration in the vitamin C content as well as the overall quality. Oranges tend to lose mass and tropical fruits tend to get soft and develop an 'off' smell. Whistle-blowers have come forward to reveal that apples in particular can stay in cold storage for up to two years.

The recommended storage times are as follows:

Apples	2-6 months
Cabbage	5-6 months
Carrots	5-9 months
Cauliflower	2-4 weeks
Leeks	1-3 months
Oranges	3-4 months
Spinach	1-2 weeks

I believe it would be reasonable to have the date of harvest displayed along with the price in order for consumers to make an informed choice. I might be motivated by the harvest date over the price if that information was readily available. I think I would pay extra for an apple that was only a few weeks old, as apposed to a couple of years old.

As if the poor fruit hadn't already been through enough, then there's the issue with artificial ripening.

The produce that is most commonly associated with artificial ripening includes bananas, mangos, strawberries, oranges, pineapple, plums, peaches, tomatoes, capsicum, cherries and coffee.

Depending on the country and the type of produce, a range of artificial ripening agents may be used. These include ethylene gas, methyl cyclopropene, calcium carbide, ethane, ethephon, bethylene, and acetylene.

There are two types of fruits, climatic and non-climatic. Climatic fruits are the tropical fruits, which will continue to ripen after picking. The non-climatic fruits, like berries will not ripen further once they have been severed from the plant. Methyl cyclopropane is used with non-climatic fruit, such as strawberries to prevent deterioration, rather than as a ripening agent.

Climatic fruit has been treated with ethylene gas for decades to ripen fruits such as bananas and tomatoes. It is actually a hormone that occurs naturally during the ripening process. The problem is, that ethylene gas is expensive. Subsequently the use of calcium carbide has taken its place. Its use was initially centred on the commercial tropical fruit industry of Bangladesh, India and Pakistan; but the use of calcium carbide has become more widespread. It is now used in Australia, South Africa, South America, China, America, Taiwan, Philippines and Malaysia. This means that most of the imported produce is artificially ripened; although in Australia its use tends to be with bananas, mangoes, tomatoes and oranges.

Calcium carbide is used, as it tends to get a good colour on the skin, making the fruit look really attractive. However, the fruit tends to stay hard and unripe on the inside. As a result, it decomposes on the inside, while looking pristine on the outside and we confuse this rotting with ripening.

If only calcium carbide was non-toxic like the ethylene gas, but it isn't. Calcium carbide when combined with the water in the fruit, forms acetylene. It may also contain traces of arsenic. It is believed to affect the nervous system by reducing oxygen to the brain. Other reported effects include: damage to the eyes, skin and lungs; memory loss; mental confusion, seizures, cerebral oedema; headaches, dizziness, mood disturbances and has strong carcinogenic properties.

Another artificial ripener is bethylene, which is less toxic but strongly affects the flavour and nutrient quality. Ethephon is another ripening agent that is in use; it has no effect on the flavour, but there is mixed reviews of its safety.

After the fruit has been ripened it generally gets dosed with propylene glycol (1520) right up until the point of sale. Those automatic mist streams that are featured in many fruit and vegetable shops are usually a propylene glycol solution, not water. Propylene glycol is a toxic chemical that is linked to neurological disorders, as well as kidney and liver damage.

The commercial fruit industry argues that artificial ripening is necessary, as ripe fruit cannot be transported without damage. It is a valid point, but the consumer has a right to know about the use of ripening agents at the point of sale. Perhaps if the type of ripening agent were advertised, people would push the market share toward the use of ethylene gas. Integrity needs to be restored to the industry. The focus is currently on appearance, longevity and profit margin. The consumer must rate a mention. The consumer is being robbed from the inherent properties of fruit and vegetables—flavour and nutrition. These are replaced with something toxic and tasteless.

There are a few solutions to reducing the presence of added chemicals. Several companies have fruit wash solutions on the market that are reputably very effective. There are also small battery operated machines that sit inside the refrigerator; they work by oxidising the air inside the fridge killing mould, bacteria and breaks down pesticide residue.

Alternatively, fruit and vegetables may be soaked in water for ten minutes before use.

Salicylates

Another consequence of artificial ripening is the accumulation of salicylates.

Salicylates are aspirin-like compounds contained in fruit and vegetables with the function of keeping the plant healthy while it is growing. Salicylate levels are at their peak during the growing phase and then decline as the ripening process completes. However, many plants will still contain salicylates in the out leaves or skin for protection, which can easily be removed.

The routine practice of picking fruit and vegetables when they are not ripe, results in unnecessarily high levels of salicylates.

Salicylates block neuro-receptors in the brain and have an accumulative effect, which makes it difficult to link the symptoms to the cause. Salicylates and commercial aspirin increases the amount of vitamin C, potassium and iron that is excreted, this can lead to lethargy and a decreased immunity. Levels can build to cause intoxication and a range of behavioural effects. We have labels for the rowdy effects, like ADHD, but it is often the quiet dreamy ones that are more affected. In my school teaching career I can attest that the children with learning difficulties tend to be the dreamy ones. Where as the disruptive children (who get more attention), tend to be quite switched on.

Interestingly, there is a lot of research into the anti-cancer properties of salicylates. Salicylates serve the function of protecting a plant against diseases. The theory is that, what is good for a plant might be good for us. So far the therapeutic effects are unproven, but the neurological effects are well established. How a person responds to salicylates is a similar to the effects of smoking. Some people can smoke a packet a day and remain largely unaffected. Other people can contract lung cancer just through passive smoking. Our constitutions are all unique. What does seem to be clear, is that children are more greatly affected due to the decreased body mass.

It is useful to do a chemical elimination diet with a salicylate challenge to assess your sensitivity to salicylates. It might be useful to ask a loved one to assess your behaviour during the challenge. If salicylates prove to be an issue, try to buy vine ripened fruit or vegetables; or better yet grow your own. Failing that, there are some commercially grown fruits and vegetables that are low in salicylates, regardless of how they are grown.

Low salicylate fruits include: pears, golden/red delicious apples, mango, persimmons, bananas, papayas, paw paw, tamarillo, rhubarb, custard apples and loquats.

Low salicylate vegetables include: lettuce, celery, green beans, peas, cabbage, brussels sprouts, garlic, potatoes, swede, butternut pumpkin, asparagus, sweet potato, choko, parsnip, spring onions, leeks, parsley, chives, sage, lentils, bamboo shoots, bean shoots and mungbean sprouts.

Most of us are aware of how important it is to eat fruit and vegetables and we do our best to get our quota. The naturally ripened, pesticide free organic produce is expensive and out of reach for most people. The average person is forced to buy the cheaper varieties of fruit or vegetables that have been stifled. We confuse rotting with ripening.

If you have you seen animals in nature, they don't select green fruit and it is usually eaten immediately. We as human beings need to get back to the practice of eating fresh produce. When fresh produce is consumed with in twenty minutes of picking, all of the live enzymes and phytochemicals are utilised. It is time to start eating as nature intended.

Get Gardening

The simplest solution to gaining access to quality, delicious and nutritious fruit and vegetables is to grow your own! Swap the flowerbed for a food garden. Most people would say that they don't have time for growing vegetables and fruit. But there is time to tend to the lawn and the petunias… We live in an age of reticulation systems. Weeding or pruning a vegetable patch is no more taxing than tending to the rose bushes.

A vegetable garden doesn't take a lot of time, but does require a consistent effort. It actually becomes quite exciting and addictive. If it really isn't your cup of tea, there are many businesses offering to do it for you and it is a lot cheaper than you might think.

As most suburban lots have an extensive history with pesticide use, I would avoid growing directly into the earth. Remember that pesticides take at least fifty years to breakdown.

Either growing in tubs or in a raised up bed is the way to go. Do spend the extra money on organic soil; after all if it's worth doing, it's worth doing properly!

You'll be amazed how satisfying it is to be self-sufficient and by the flavour difference. Try to stagger what you are growing so that it doesn't all ripen at once. In other words don't plant all of your tomatoes at the same time, spread it out over a few weeks and the harvest time will last longer. Broccoli is a vegetable I have grown at home and when it's produced with out chemicals, it goes limp very fast after harvesting, it always amazes me how long the commercially grown ones last!

There are a few options when you have an abundance of something. You can blanch and freeze if it is appropriate; make a puree cooked or uncooked and place it in the freezer for up to three months; invest in a dehydrator; or give the extras to your nearests and dearests.

Research has showed that kids love getting dirty and are more likely to try something new if they have been involved in its care and production. In my experience from being a schoolteacher and a mother, planting seeds and nurturing seedlings is really rewarding. I am yet to discover a child who doesn't experience a genuine thrill when the seeds first shoot; when the first flower appears; or proudly presenting their ripe produce to their loved ones.

Gardening doesn't have to be expensive. Just about anything can be recycled to raise seedlings in and people use all sorts of things as garden pots; if it can hold soil, it can be transformed into a pot. Instead of throwing the pips in the bin, try building a seed bank by saving and drying seeds. In addition, many varieties can be grown from cuttings.

Seasonal Eating

There was once a time when the availability of fruit and vegetable varieties were dependent on the season. With the onset of long-term cold storage, hydroponics and globalisation, almost everything is available all year round. I believe this system defies nature. What if there is a purpose to eating with divine timing? Even if you can't stretch that far, eating seasonally will increase the likelihood of fruit or vegetable's freshness. Of course if you embrace the joy of gardening, divine law must reign and knowledge of the seasons is key.

Kylie Floate

Summer harvest

Asparagus
Tomatoes
Green beans
Egg plant
Broccoli
Capsicum
Corn
Leek
Cucumber
Parsnip
Silverbeet
Zucchini
Rockmelon
Watermelon
Honeydew melon
Peaches
Nectarines
Cherries

Autumn Harvest

Pumpkin
Broccoli
Brussels sprouts
Capsicum
Celery
Corn
Eggplant
Kale
Leek
Cucumber
Parsnip
Peas
Silverbeet
Swede
Tomato

Zucchini
Rockmelon
Watermelon
Honeydew melon
Grapes

Winter Harvest

Pumpkin
Broad Beans
Cauliflower
Celery
Parsnip
Peas
Swede
Oranges
Apples
Pears
Persimmons

Spring Harvest

Leek
Cauliflower
Peas
Zucchini (late)
Apples
Oranges
Pears

Perennial

Lettuce
Most Herbs
Beetroot
Cabbage
Carrots
Chilli
Onion

Phase Four—
Balancing the pH of Food

Tradition meets western science

The pH scale is a measure of the acidity or alkalinity of a substance. It ranges from 0-14, with 7 classed as neutral. The lower end of the scale is acidic and the upper end alkaline. The body's homeostasis is 7.4, which is slightly alkaline. Foods are can be categorised as acidic or alkaline according to how they affect the pH of urine.

For thousands of years the eating habits of many cultures have been affected by the 'heating' and 'cooling' affect of food. The 'heating' refers to acidic foods and the 'cooling' refers to alkaline foods. This practice has its roots from Ayurvedia, Chinese medicine and allopathy, but has also become very popular within the New Age movement.

Until recently, there was no separation between nutrition and medicine. Examination of the food intake was routinely used to treat illness. The rise of pharmaceuticals in the Western world led to a declined interest in nutrition. The magic pill has great appeal! The use of multivitamins and a course of antibiotics have replaced proper nutrition, drinking water, exercise and getting sufficient sleep. However, in Asia, the Middle East, Mediterranean Europe and the developing world a traditional approach to medicine is the first port of call.

Ayurveda

Ayurveda is synonymous with Indian culture and its antiquity goes back to the Vedas five thousand years ago. Ayurveda is the Sanskrit word for "scripture for longevity" or "life and knowledge". It is based on creating a state of equilibrium within the mind, body, soul and intellect. The philosophy is based on the understanding that positive health is influenced by diet, state of mind (consciousness), environment and lifestyle factors.

The emphasis is placed on prevention. There are different dietary and lifestyle recommendations for each season. Often herbal remedies are ingested for the prevention of disease, purification or rejuvenation. Other times they are prescribed therapeutically to treat disease.

All conditions are considered potentially treatable and the treatment of the disease is highly individual. All physical, emotional, psychological, behavioural, spiritual, material and environmental aspects of an individual's life are taken into consideration. Meditation and yoga are almost always part of the prescription.

Conventional Western research is flimsy. The studies are largely centred around the use of herbal remedies without taking into account the entire scope of the treatment. Indian research takes a comprehensive approach and has found considerable data showing the efficacy of Ayurveda in treating diabetes, neuro-degenerative disorders, heart disease and anxiety reduction.

Allopathy

Allopathy stems from Ayurvedic medicine and is an ancient practice of 'opposites'. In the middle ages it was the most widespread form of medicine.

Food, diseases and body parts are described as being 'hot' or 'cold'. Imbalance is said to be the cause of all disease. A patient is assessed by clinical signs and symptoms; behaviour; environmental conditions and diet composition. Imbalance can occur in one or more areas.

In addition to the hot or cold valence that is assigned to the food, the elements of earth, air, fire, water and ether also play a role. Each correspond to the taste sensations of sweet, sour, salty, pungent, bitter and astringent.

The season of harvest, stage of ripeness, water content and mode of preparation are also taken into consideration in relation to its heating and cooling effects. Foods are also said to produce different moods and behaviours. Overall, allopathy is much more food based than spiritual.

Chinese Medicine

Chinese medicine involves a yin/yang philosophy, Yin is female, and it represents cold, dark and wet. Yang is male which represents light, dry and hot. All foods are classified as hot, cold or neutral and like allopathy it is aligned with the elements, except that wood substitutes ether.

Chinese medicine has all the hallmarks of allopathy and Ayurveda, but also incorporates astrology and works more on a continuum. In other words, rather than a food classified as a static hot or cold substance, it is described as weakly or strongly hot or cold.

Cravings for flavours play an important role in the diagnosis of disease. Chinese medicine is one of the most carefully balanced, complex systems. It also has homeopathic similarities, where a little 'poison' is administrated to treat to disease as like dissolves in like.

Scientific evidence

A highly acidic diet is linked to osteoporosis, heart disease, a variety of cancers, Parkinson's disease, aging and illness. This seems to be caused by a mechanism that draws minerals from the bone and soft tissue in order to maintain the body's pH. On the other hand, an alkaline diet seems to keep the body oxygenated and running optimally.

An average adult consuming a Western diet generates 50-100mEq acid/day. This level is classified as chronic low-grade acidosis. Bone in particular, acts as a buffer by delivering calcium ions, but over time this process leads to the dissolution of bone minerals and bone density. As age progresses, this mechanism also results in declined kidney function.

One study of healthy adults given an acidic diet showed a 74% increase in calcium excretion compared to when they were given an alkaline diet.

Several studies have found that excess acid intake through the diet is a risk factor for oesteoporosis and that diets rich in potassium and bicarbonates, namely fruit and vegetables, are highly correlated with increased bone density.

A double-blind study of young women found that drinking calcium-rich water had no affect on bone resorption, whereas, alkaline bicarbonate rich water strongly affected bone resorption.

A large study conducted by Cambridge University, found that women were much more susceptible to the adverse effects of an acidic diet when compared to men. The same study also confirmed that an acidic diet was associated with decreased bone density.

Another recent study by Cambridge University (2010), found that water consumption greatly affects the acid/alkaline balance. Other studies have found that the temperature that a person bathes or showers in also affects the body's pH. Hot showers are associated with increased acidity.

How to create a PH balance

The extreme approach would be mostly concerned with the overall pH balance of the body. This would involve separating acidic and alkaline foods, as consuming them together alters the overall pH. However, I believe that a more sensible approach is advisable. Aim for 80% alkaline forming foods and 20% acidic foods. Opt for a diet that is rich in alkaline fruit and vegetables, along with the weakly acidic wholegrain foods. Follow a meal with 'cooling' alkaline foods like a lovely piece a fruit. The message here is raising awareness that the average Western person consumes a highly acidic diet consisting of meat, dairy, cereal, bread, pasta, rice, processed foods and alcohol. Small changes can achieve an optimal body pH and drastically reduce the risk factor for various diseases.

Table of Acidic and Alkaline foods

Alkaline foods

Alfalfa	Parsley
Almonds	Avocado
Asparagus	Barley
Broccoli	Beetroot (fresh)
Beans	Brussels sprouts
Cabbage	Cauliflower
Chestnuts	Celery
Cucumber	Capsicum
Carrots	Dandelion
Eggplant	Garlic
Hazelnut	Kale
Lettuce	Lentils
Mushroom	Peas
Potatoes	Pumpkin
Okra	Onion
Radish	Seaweed
Silverbeet	Squash
Sweet potato	Tomato
Turnip	Watercress
Wild rice	Apples
Apricot	Banana
Cherries	Citrus fruit
Coconut	Dates
Grapes	Grapefruit
Figs	Honeydew melon
Kiwifruit	Mango
Nectarine	Pear
Peach	Pineapple
Raison	Rhubarb
Rockmelon	Sultanas
Watermelon	Pumpkin seeds

Sunflower seeds

Black strap molasses

Curry spices

Ginger

Goat cheese

Probiotic cultures

Tempeh

Canola oil

Olive oil

Sugar

Apple cider vinegar

Cinnamon

Turmeric

Sea salt

Natural yoghurt

Tofu

Tea (black, green and herbal)

Grapeseed oil

Unsalted butter

Acidic foods

Meat

Animal derived products

Eggs

Pasta

Blueberries

Plums

Cashew nuts

Walnuts

Alcohol

Dairy foods

Seafood

Bread

Rice

Cranberries

Prunes

Pistachios

Honey

Wheat-based products

Whole grains including oats, corn, quinoa, amaranth

Phase Five—Conscious eating

Environmental and health implications of food

It might surprise you to learn that a vegan diet is in fact the most healthy. Scientific evidence now confirms that diets high in animal products are highly correlated with the prevalence of chronic diseases. A vegan diet is one that is plant-based and excludes the consumption of all animal products.

Vegan diets tend to be low in cholesterol and total fat, high in fibre, phytochemicals, antioxidants (particularly vitamin C and E), folic acid and magnesium. Studies have shown vegan diets are beneficial in the prevention and treatment of cardiovascular disease, hypertension, coronary heart disease, type 2 diabetes, cancer, osteoporosis, kidney disease, dementia, Parkinson's disease, rheumatoid arthritis, gallstones and diverticular disease.

Until recently, a vegan diet was considered potentially deficient of iron, vitamin B12 and zinc. While it is true that stores of those nutrients do tend to be lower, there is now evidence that lower iron stores may actually reduce the risk of chronic disease. Non-haem iron also seems to be absorbed more efficiently in the absence of haem-iron. Meaning that the body becomes lazy in the presence of the readily absorbed haem-iron, but is actually quite capable of absorbing non-haem iron effectively. Vitamin B12 has been found to be the most highly efficiently recycled vitamin. Deficiency would take up to ten years to set in. Zinc is found in legumes, cereals and nuts—a carefully planned vegan diet can provide the RDIs.

Vegans tend to be leaner, with a low BMI, lower rates of chronic disease and increased longevity. It is the position of the American Dietetic Association (A.D.A.) that a vegan diet, when planned well are *"healthful, nutritionally adequate and may provide health benefits in the prevention and treatment of certain diseases"* In addition, the A.D.A. has deemed a vegan diet as appropriate for all stages of life, including pregnancy, lactating, infancy, childhood, adolescence and even athletes.

The employees of a major insurance company participated in a recent study (2010) to explore the effects of a vegan diet on health and work productivity for twenty-two weeks.

The participants had a BMI of 25 or greater and/or a previous type two diabetes diagnosis. The vegan group reported improvement in their general health, physical functioning, mental health, vitality and decreased food cost, but reported difficulty finding food when eating out compared to the control group. There were 46% fewer sick days in the vegan group than the control group. They concluded that a vegan diet could improve the quality of life and work productivity of the employees.

Other research has shown that a vegan diet leads to a rapid remission in the complications associated with type two diabetes. These complications include glycaemia (blood sugar level), neuropathic pain (caused by loss of sensation in the extremities) and obesity. The American Diabetes Council now recommends a vegan diet after studies showed greater improvements on a vegan diet, than diets based on more conventional guidelines.

Cambridge University (2005) performed one of the several studies that indicated a vegan diet is particularly beneficial in the prevention and management of osteoporosis.

Another study conducted in 2009, indicated that twenty-nine other randomised control trials concluded that a vegan diet had the greatest influence on lowering blood lipid levels and producing overall weight loss.

Vegetarians who eat a grain and dairy based diet have been found to have the same risk of disease as non-vegetarians. The consumption of dairy products is associated with a higher risk of colorectal cancer, prostate cancer, ovarian cancer and breast cancer. The interesting fact is that approximately 15% of the world's population (mostly Caucasian) possess the enzyme lactase, which is necessary to breakdown lactose in milk after the age of four. Which means that at least 85% of the Western population is likely to be lactose intolerant. Asian people are notorious for their avoidance of dairy products, favouring soy instead. Approximately 98% of Indigenous Australians are lactose intolerant and having had direct observation, I can attest that there seems to be little awareness of this fact among the people.

Many cultures breastfeed their infants until the age of 5, with water substituted beyond that. The concept of drinking another animal's milk is foreign to many around the world. Dairy products are also high in phenylalanine.

Phenylalanine is an amino acid that is found in dairy and as an additive to several diet beverages and food products. It is a particularly important amino acid for cows and has a tendency to accumulate in the body. Babies are tested at birth during the Guthrie's heal prick test to determine if phenylalanine can be metabolised at all. A person does not need to have Phenylketonuria (PKU) in order to experience adverse effects. A dairy intolerance can often be difficulties with phenylalanine.

Phenylalanine reduces the rate at which protein is synthesised in the brain, resulting in impaired mental function and in severe cases, causes mental retardation. Mild symptoms are associated with gastrointestinal function, like wind and diarrhoea.

Much of the world practices vegetarianism or veganism, usually for religious or cultural reasons. However, there are a growing number of people who convert to a vegan lifestyle for moral, ethical and environmentally sustainable reasons. When one considers the conditions of the feedlot or the conventions of abattoirs it is easy to see why. Commercial slaughterhouses are not pretty. Somehow our culture has become desensitised to the reality of it all. Meat has become just another item at the supermarket. I wonder how many people would actually have the stomach to slaughter an animal. If the middleman were cut out of the equation, how many people would suddenly turn vegan?

The livestock industry is one of the largest contributors to environmental degradation. In Australia, salinity is a serious issue. Mass land clearing for agricultural purposes is the main cause of salinity. The impact on ecosystems and species numbers has been considerable. Beef production has been widely cited as the driving force behind the destruction of the Amazon rainforest and other key ecological areas.

Livestock production requires ten times more water than a grain crop, plus more grain per hectare to feed the animals than what the land could ordinarily produce.

In fact it takes 20,000 litres or 5283 gallons of water to produce 1 kilogram or 2lbs of beef. Additionally, each cow chews its way through approximately 100 kg or 220lbs of food in order to produce 1kg or 2.2lbs of beef.

The requirements of beef production are three times that of pork or lamb and about four times that of chicken. A chicken requires 87 litres or 23 gallons of water and 4.5 kg or 10lbs of grain in order to produce 1kg or 2.2lbs of meat or eggs.

The director of the centre for global food issues recently stated *"the world must create 5 billion vegans in the next several decades, or triple its total farm output without using more land"*. Hence the introduction of the feedlot operation.

In Belgium, they have introduced weekly meat free days and imposed vegetarian only meals for canteens catering to civil servants and schools. Instead of taking a cue from Belgium, the world's hope for future meat consumption is pinned on invitro or cultured meat. Invitro meat is artificially synthesised muscle fibre produced in laboratories. Not only does it give new meaning to the concept of Frankenstein food, but also it is estimated to double the cost of meat in the future.

If going vegan is a bit of a stretch for you at this time, do consider regular meat free days, or maybe make a vegetarian lunch. We all have to start somewhere!

Food sources and nutrient intake

There are many nutrients that we are conditioned to believe come only from animal products. The following is a list of fruit, vegetable and nut or seed sources of iron, calcium, zinc and Vitamin B12 per 100g.

Iron

Fruit Sources:	Raisins	4.2 mg
	Apricots	3.1 mg
	Dates	2.6 mg
	Mango	2.5 mg
	Sultanas	2.0 mg
	Pineapple	1.9 mg
	Cherries	1.6 mg
	Figs	1.4 mg
	Blueberries	1.3 mg
	Strawberries	1.3 mg
	Peaches	1.2 mg
	Prunes	1.1 mg
	Bananas	1.1 mg
Vegetable Sources:	seaweed	14.6mg
	Parsley	9.4 mg
	Beancurd/tofu	7.9 mg
	Lentils	7.5 mg
	Potatoes	7.0 mg
	Haricot beans	6.4 mg
	Tomatoes	5.4 mg
	Peas	3.8 mg
	Broccoli	3.6 mg
	Spinach	3.2 mg
	Kale	3.1 mg
	Watercress	3.0 mg
	Chives	2.8 mg
	Chickpeas	2.5 mg
	Dried beans	2.4 mg
	Vine leaves	2.3 mg
	Snow peas	2.3 mg
	Silverbeet	2.1 mg
	Onion	2.1 mg
	Horseradish	2.0 mg
	Cabbage	1.7 mg
	Garlic	1.7 mg
	Asparagus	1.6 mg

Chicory	1.6 mg
Rocket	1.5 mg
Beetroot	1.3 mg
Bok choy	1.3 mg
Chilli	1.3 mg
Capsicum	1.1 mg
Green beans	1.1 mg
Lettuce	1.1 mg

Nut and Seed Sources:

Tahini	15.5mg
Pumpkin seeds	10.0mg
Poppy seeds	8.7 mg
Cashews	6.3 mg
Sunflower seeds	4.5 mg
Pistachios	4.2 mg
Pine nuts	4.1 mg
Almonds	3.6 mg
Hazelnuts	3.3 mg
Peanuts	2.4 mg
Pecans	2.4 mg
Walnuts	2.3 mg
Brazil nuts	2.2 mg
Macadamias	1.8 mg

Calcium

Fruit Sources:

Figs	200 mg
Pineapple	168 mg
Orange peel	161 mg
Lemon peel	161 mg
Apricots	67 mg
Currants	87 mg
Sultanas	56 mg
Prunes	52 mg
Dates	47 mg
Nectarines	47 mg
Kumquats	44 mg
Honeydew melon	39 mg

	Peach	37 mg
	Mango	35 mg
	Banana	32 mg
	Blackberry	30 mg
	Persimmon	29 mg
	Kiwi fruit	29 mg
	Plums	29 mg
	Paw paw	28 mg
	Logan berries	28 mg
	Mandarins	26 mg
	Cherries	26 mg
	Raspberries	23 mg
	Tangelos	22 mg
	Grapefruit	21 mg
	Mulberries	20 mg
	Jackfruit	18 mg
	Rhubarb	18 mg
	Apple	18 mg
	Custard apple	17 mg
	Boysenberries	15 mg
	Strawberries	14 mg
	Green grapes	12 mg
Vegetable Sources:	Seaweed	663 mg
	Soybeans	450 mg
	Vine leaves	384 mg
	Bean curd/tofu	336 mg
	Mushrooms	319 mg
	Onion	239 mg
	Basil	230 mg
	Parsley	200 mg
	Broccoli	196 mg
	English spinach	170 mg
	Potato	165 mg
	Rocket	160 mg
	Cauliflower	160 mg
	Kale	154 mg
	Haricot beans	150 mg

Horseradish	120 mg
Zucchini	115 mg
Tomato	97 mg
Chives	90 mg
Watercress	85 mg
Okra	78 mg
Lentils	73 mg
Cabbage	70 mg
Borlotti beans	70 mg
Silverbeet	68 mg
Cucumber	63 mg
Bok choy	60 mg
Peas	42 mg
Celery	42 mg
Pumpkin	36 mg
Parsnip	36 mg
Red kidney beans	35 mg
Sweet potato	35 mg
Red cabbage	35 mg
Carrot	34 mg
Artichoke	33 mg
Leek	33 mg
Green beans	33 mg
Garlic	30 mg
Chicory	29 mg
Radish	25 mg
Eggplant	24 mg
Spring onion	22 mg
Chilli	22 mg
Swede	21 mg
Turnip	21 mg
Chinese cabbage	21 mg
Fennel	20 mg
Lettuce	20 mg
Avocado	20 mg
Alfalfa	19 mg
Choko	17 mg

	Lima beans	15 mg
	Butter beans	15 mg
	Bamboo shoots	15 mg
	Marrow	15 mg
	Brussels sprout	15 mg
	Squash	9 mg
	Beetroot	8 mg
	Capsicum	8 mg
	Corn	4 mg
	Shitake mushrooms	4 mg
Nut and Seed Sources:	Poppy seeds	1448 mg
	Sesame paste	744 mg
	Almonds	339 mg
	Brazil nuts	150 mg
	Sunflower seeds	100 mg
	Pistachios	97 mg
	Hazelnuts	90 mg
	Walnuts	89 mg
	Peanuts	55 mg
	Pecans	51 mg
	Macadamias	48 mg
	Chestnuts	39 mg
	Pumpkin seeds	39 mg
	Cashews	35 mg
	Pine nuts	11 mg

Zinc

Fruit Sources:	Mango	1.5 mg
	Pineapple	1.2 mg
Vegetable Sources:	Tomato	13.6mg
	Seaweed	4.8 mg
	Lentils	3.0 mg
	Peas	2.4 mg
	Dried beans	2.4 mg
	Mushrooms	2.3 mg
	Vine leaves	1.9 mg

	Onion	1.8 mg
	Soybeans	1.6 mg
	Cabbage	1.5 mg
	Green beans	1.4 mg
	Horseradish	1.4 mg
	Capsicum	1.4 mg
	Parsley	1.2 mg
	Bean curd/tofu	1.2 mg
	Bamboo shoots	1.1 mg
	Potato	1.1 mg
Nut and Seed Sources:	Poppy seeds	10.2 mg
	Pumpkin seeds	6.6 mg
	Sunflower seeds	6.5 mg
	Cashews	5.7 mg
	Sesame seeds	5.5 mg
	Tahini	5.2 mg
	Brazil nuts	4.1 mg
	Pecans	3.9 mg
	Almonds	3.8 mg
	Walnuts	2.5 mg
	Pistachios	2.5 mg
	Hazelnuts	2.3 mg
	Macadamias	1.2 mg

Vitamin B12

The main plant based source of vitamin B12 is mushrooms. However, there is evidence that B12 is synthesised by bacteria living on the surface of fruit and vegetables. B12 will only be eliminated if thorough washing of the fruit or vegetable prior to consumption occurs.

I recommend a feed of mushrooms every couple of months. As I am not a big fan of mushrooms, I find that they can be blended and added to sauces quite easily. If you happen to like mushrooms, then there is really no need to worry about developing a vitamin B12 deficiency.

Suggested Meal Plans

Veganism must be approached consciously, ensuring that the nutrient intake is adequate. The first thing I would do is to purchase a few vegan cookbooks. Get some recipes in your repertoire and build your confidence. Cooking with unfamiliar items or in brand new ways can be a bit daunting at first. Learn from others and get a sense of what flavours go together before you try to be creative. Try not to cook your old favourites minus the meat; as it leaves one feeling short changed. Be adventurous!

A basic meal plan would look something like this:

Breakfast:	Porridge made with oats, quinoa or amaranth
	Muesli
	Cereal
	Fruit smoothie
	Vegan loaf
	Toast
Morning/Afternoon Tea:	Dried/fresh fruit
	Nuts
	Biscuits or similar
Lunch:	Salad
	Sandwich
	Hummus/tabouli with crackers and veggie sticks
	Felafal kebab
	Soup and bread
Dinner:	Indian cuisine
	Risotto
	Pilaf
	Pasta
	Stir fries with rice, noodles, quinoa or couscous
	Vegetable patties with salad or vegetables
	Felafals
	Savoury crepes

Dessert:

Pies and pastries
Tacos and nachos
Fresh/ steamed/dried fruit
Dairy free ice cream
Fruit sorbet
Fruit crumble
Bean curd desserts
Indian desserts
/semolina/taro cakes

Phase Six—Food Integrity

Utilising the life force in food

Inside all livings things there is a spark of life, including plants. When a fruit or vegetable is harvested, it continues to respire. What it is actually doing is breathing out very slowly. The time it takes for a fruit or vegetable to expire depends on the variety. Something with a soft exterior, like a strawberry will die quickly, within a few days. Something with a hard exterior, like a pumpkin, will live for several months. Keeping the roots and outer leaves intact will help with preservation.

Ultimately, when the flesh of a fruit or vegetable is cut into or cooked, the life force will expire within about twenty minutes. Many of the live enzymes, phytochemicals, flavonoids and antioxidants are also destroyed in this timeframe. In order to utilise the life force and the additional components within the produce, it is important to buy whole items, uncut. Try to incorporate plenty of raw food in your diet that is consumed within that twenty minute time period. Sometimes this isn't always practical, some people just wouldn't use a whole watermelon or cabbage. Food wastage and cash expenditure are just as serious issues.

Gratitude and savouring the moment

My first attempts at 'feeling gratitude' left me feeling ridiculous. At school we were forced to say grace before we could go out to lunch. This was usually met with eye rolling, smirks and going through the motions to get it over with. Some of my friends' parents insisted on saying grace when I went for a sleepover. I always felt embarrassed, like my family was beneath them as we weren't deeply religious. The grace that I witnessed appeared to be done out of god-fearing, as though they would burn in hell if the words weren't uttered. I didn't see a lot of actual gratitude.

The kind of gratitude I am referring to is appreciation. Taking the time to appreciate what was involved to grow the things that are intended for your meal. The average food crop takes five months to ripen, some are ready in a few short months and others might take nine months. Many vegetables are dependant on the presence of frost and then the sun blooming at precisely the right time. Many fruit and nuts trees take two to three years to reach fruit baring maturity. Many varieties take several years to get properly established and produce high yields.

When I was a child, we planted a macadamia nut tree as a seedling. We lovingly nurtured it for two years before the first blossoms appeared. Only a handful of the blossoms turned into nuts. The excitement we had tasting these first nuts was immense. The gratitude and appreciation we had for our macadamia tree was wonderful.

As I write this, I am living in rural Western Australia. This is an area that is known for its crops of wheat, oats, barley and canola. The nine months it takes from seed to harvest is a real roller coaster ride. The hopes and prayers the farmers have for ideal weather is overwhelming. If a bout of unexpected weather threatens the crops it is all anyone in the community will talk about. It is their livelihood and the community really bands together when times are tough. Likewise, harvest time is a time of genuine celebration. The community feels gratitude (and a little relief)!

The gratitude and appreciation seems to end there. It then becomes just another commodity to buy and consume, with the attitude that 'there's plenty more where that came from'.

By now you should have experienced the satisfaction that comes from producing some of your own food. It is easy to experience gratitude and appreciation when you are consuming the fruits of your labour. Even if something isn't homegrown, the gratitude should not lessen. The plant still had to survive by the grace of God for many months before reaching your plate. Many of the nut, fruit, vegetable and grain crops come from poor countries, where growers are paid very little and must work in extreme conditions.

Instead of wolfing down your meal without a second thought, take a moment to appreciate the food for all that it is and how it came to be. Thank God for providing the conditions that allowed it to thrive and that it is destined for your stomach. Hunger and deprivation are not something that we in the developed world usually experience. Take a moment to feel grateful that starvation is not apart of your reality. Gratitude doesn't need to be a vocal act; just a moment silently will suffice. Ensure that it is sincere, if it is only done out of obligation there really is no point.

Here are some everyday foods and their usual growing periods.

Apples:	2 years to bare fruit, then one crop seasonally
Pears:	5 years to bare fruit, then one crop seasonally
Peaches:	1 year to bare fruit, then one crop seasonally
Nectarines:	1 year to bare fruit, then one crop seasonally
Grapes:	2 years to first harvest, then one crop seasonally
Rockmelon:	4 months
Asparagus:	2-3 years for the first crop
Broad beans:	3 months
Green beans:	3 months
Lettuce:	2-3 months
Carrots:	5 months
Tomatoes:	4 months
Cucumbers:	3-4 months
Cabbage:	4 months
Potatoes:	5-9 months
Parsnip:	5 months
Celery:	4 months
Capsicum:	3 months
Broccoli:	3 months
Brussels sprouts:	3 months

Cauliflower:	5 months
Leek:	4 months
Onions:	9 months
Chilli:	3 months
Beetroot:	3 months
Peas:	3 months
Zucchini:	2 months
Silverbeet:	3 months
Swede:	3 months
Corn:	3 months
Kale:	2 months
Pumpkin:	6 months
Eggplant:	4 months

Embracing a New Future

Be a shiny example for others to follow. Instead of whinging about everything, be the change that you would like to see in the world. Change is a gradual process, an evolution. There are always the early adopters and the laggards. It is far more productive to focus on what we can change rather than what we can't.

In terms of the food supply, I firmly believe that everything comes down to market share and economics. Simply choose items that are produced ethically. Collectively, we can assert change. Sign on to petitions that lobby disclosure and safety in our food supply, or write to your member of parliament. The current approach to food production will only continue if we accept it. Go on I dare you!

References

Allen, D.H., Van Nunens, S., Loblay, R., Clark, L. & Swain, A. (1984). Adverse reactions to foods, *Medical Journal Australia;* 141(S37-S42)

Ashraf-Ur-Rahman, F.R.Chowdhury, & B. Alam. (2008). Artificial ripening: what are we eating. *Journal of Medicine*; (9): 42-44.

Barker, A. (1975). Organic vs inorganic nutrition and horticultural crop quality. *Horticultural Science;* 10: pp. 50-53.

Bateman, B., Warner, J., Hutchinson, E. et al. (2004). The effects of double blind, placebo controlled artificial food colourings and benzoate preservative challenge on hyperactivity on the general population: sample of preschool children. *Archives of Disabled Children;* 89: 506-11.

Ball, M. (1997). Diabetes. Wahlqvist, M.L. (Ed.), *Allen & Unwin, Australia.*

Barnard, N.D., Scialli, A.R., Turner-McGrievy, G., H. (2004). Acceptability of low-fat vegan diet compares favourably to a step II diet in a randomised controlled diet. *Journal of cardiopulmonary rehabilitation.* July-Aug; 24(4): pp. 229-235.

Barnard, N.D., Cohen, J., Jenkins, D.J., Turner-McGrievy, G., Gloede, L., Jaster, B., Seidl, K., Green, A., Talpers, S. (2006). A low-fat vegan diet improves glycaemic control and cardiovascular risk factors in a randomised clinical trial in individuals with type 2 diabetes. *Diabetes care.* Aug; 29(8): pp. 1777-1783.

Barnard, N.D., Cohen, J., Jenkins, D.J., Turner-McGrievy, G., Gloede, L., Green, A. Ferdowsian, H. (2009). A low-fat diet elicits greater macronutrient changes, but is comparable in adherence and acceptability, compared with a more conventional diabetes diet among individuals with type 2 diabetes. *The American journal of clinical nutrition.*Feb; 109(2): pp. 263-273.

Barnard, N.D., Cohen, J., Jenkins, D.J., Turner-McGrievy, G., Gloede, L., Green, A. Ferdowsian, H. (2009). A low-fat vegan diet and conventional diabetes diet in the treatment of type 2 diabetes: a randomised, controlled 74-week clinical trial. *The American journal of clinical nutrition.* May; 89(5): pp 1588S-1596S.

Briggs, D.R. (1997). Food additives. Wahlqvist, M.L. (Ed.), *Allen & Unwin, Australia.*

Briggs, D.R. (1997). Naturally occurring toxicants and food contaminants. Wahlqvist, M.L. (Ed.), *Allen & Unwin, Australia.*

Briggs, D.R. & Lennard, L.B. (1997). Recent developments in food technologies. (In). Food and Nutrition. Wahlqvist, M.L. (Ed.), *Allen & Unwin, Australia.*

Chan, E., Griffiths, S., & Chan, C. (2008). Public health risks of melamine in milk products. *Lancet; 372.*

Cobiac, L. (1994). Lactose: A review of intakes and of importance of health of Australians and New Zealanders. *Supplement to Food Australia*; 46(1-28)

Craig, W.J., Mangels, A.R., American Dietetic Association. (2009). Position of the American Dietetic Association: vegetarian diets. *Journal of the American Dietetic Association.* July; 109(7): pp. 1266-1282.

David, T.J. (1993). *Food additive intolerance in childhood.* Blackwell Scientific Publications, London.

Davis, D.R. (2009). Declining fruit and vegetable nutrient composition: what is the evidence? *Horticultural Science*; 44(1)pp.15-19.

Dengate, S. (2008). *Fed up.* Random House, NSW

Dwer, J. (1999). Convergence of plant-rich and plant only diets. *American journal of clinical nutrition.* Sept; 70(3 suppl): pp. 620S-622S.

Editorial. (2007). Food safety reforms in the USA. *The Lancet;* 369: 12/05/07.

Eady, J. (2008). *Additive alert.* Additive Alert, WA.

Elder, C. (2004). Ayurveda for diabetes mellitus: a review of biomedical literature. *Alternative therapies for health and medicine: January-February 10(1) pp. 44-50.*

Epstein, S. (2002). *Unreasonable risk.* Environmental toxicology, Illinois.

Fieldhouse, P. (2002). Food and nutrition. *Nelson Thornes, UK.*

Feingold, B.F. (1975). Hyperkinesis and learning disabilities linked to artificial food colours and flavours. *American Journal of Nursing; 75:* pp.797-803.

Ferdowsian, H.R., Barnard, N.D. (2009). Effects of plant-based diets on plasma lipids. *The American journal of cardiology.* Oct; 104(7): pp. 947-956.

Fergusson, J. *The vitamin murders.* Portebello Books, London.

Jones, G.P. (1997). Food processing. (In). Wahlqvist, M.L. (Ed.), *Allen & Unwin, Australia.*

Jones, G.P. (1997). Minerals. (In). Wahlqvist, M.L. (Ed.), *Allen & Unwin, Australia.*

Jones, G.P. (1997). Water. (In). Wahlqvist, M.L. (Ed.), *Allen & Unwin, Australia.*

Hoeksma, M., Reijngould, D.J., & Pruim, J. et al. (2009). Phenylketonuria: High plasma phenylalanine decreases cerebral protein synthesis. *Journal of Molecular Genetic Metabolism;* 5/2/09

Katcher, H.I., Ferdowsian, H.R., Hoover, V.J., Cohen, J.L., Barnard, N.D. (2010). A worksite vegan nutrition program is well-accepted and improves health-related quality of life and work productivity. *Annuals of nutrition and metabolism.* 56(4): pp. 245-252.

Kennedy, E.T., Bowman, S.A., Spence, J.T., Freedmen, M., King, J. (2001) Popular diets: correlation to health, nutrition and obesity. *Journal of American Dietetic Association.* April; 101(4): pp. 411- 420.

Lau, K. (2005). Synergistic interactions between commonly used food additives in a developmental neurotoxicity test. *Toxicology Science (12)*

Leitzmann, C. (2005). Vegetarian diets: what are the advantages? *Forum of nutrition.* (57): pp. 147-156.

Loblay, R. & Swain, A.R. (1996). Food intolerance. In *Recent Advances in Clinical Nutrition 2.* Wahlqvist, M.L. & Truswell, A.S. (eds). John Libbey, London.

Loewenberg, S. (2008). US to debate tightening legislation on safety of chemicals. *Lancet;* 372: 23-24.

Marntani, R. (2005). Ayurveda and yoga in cardiovascular diseases. *Cardiology in review; May-June, 13(3): pp. 155-162.*

Mayer, A.M. (1997). Historical changes in mineral content of fruits and vegetables: a cause for concern. *British Food Journal;* 99: pp.207-11.

McCann, D., & Barrett, A. et al. (2007). Food additives and hyperactive behaviour in 3 year olds and 8/9 year old children in the community: a randomised, double blinded placebo controlled trial. *Lancet; 370* pp.1560-67.

McCarty, M.F. (1999). Vegan proteins may reduce risk of cancer, obesity, and cardiovascular disease by promoting increased glucagon activity. *Medical hypotheses.* Dec; 53(6): pp. 459-485.

McCarty, M.F. (2001). Does a vegan diet reduce risk for Parkinson's disease? *Medical hypotheses.* Sept; 57(3): pp. 318-323.

McCarty, M.F. (2002). Favourable impact of a vegan diet with exercise on herorheology: implications for control of diabetic neuropathy. *Medical hypotheses.*June; 58(6): pp. 476-486.

Messina, V., Melina, V., Mangels, A.R. (2003). A new food guide for vegetarians. *Canadian jouranal of dietetics and practical research.* 64(2): pp. 82-86.

Millstone, E. Lang, T. (2008). Risking regulatory capture at the UK's Food Standards Agency? *The Lancet; 372:* 12/07.08

Mishra,L., Sinngh, B. B., Dagenais, S. (2001). Ayurveda: a historical perspective and principles of the traditional healthcare system in India. *Alternative therapies in health and medicine.* March;7(2): pp.36-42.

N.a. (2009). Evidence on declining fruit and vegetable nutrient composition. *U.S. Food Policy.* 3/2/09.

N.a.(1983). Final report on the safety assessment of sodium lauryl sulphate. *Journal of the American College of Toxicology;*2(7).

Na. (2009). Food safety, food additives. *Centre for science in the public interest.*

Overmeyers, S. & Taylor, E. (1999). Annotation: principles of treatment for hyperkinetic disorders, practice approaches for the UK. *Journal of Child Psychology and Psychiatry;* 40: pp 1147-57.

Perry, J. (2008). China's tainted infant formula sickens nearly 13,000 babies. *British Medical Journal; 337.*

Read, R.S.D. Jones, G.P. (1997). Food energy and energy expenditure. (In). Wahlqvist, M.L. (Ed.), *Allen & Unwin, Australia.*

Sabate, J. (2003). The contribution of vegetarian diets to human health. *Forum of nutrition; 56: pp. 218-220.*

Sabate, J. Wien, M. (2010). Vegetarian diets and childhood obesity prevention. *The American journal of clinical nutrition.* May; 91(5): 1525S-1529S.

Saha, P.R, Trumbo, P.R. (1996). The nutritional adequacy of a limited vegan diet for a controlled ecological life-support system. *Advances in space research: the official journal of the committee on space research.* 18(4-5): pp.63-72.

Salisbury, F.B., Clark, M.A. (1996). Suggestions for crops grown in controlled ecological life-support systems, based on attractive vegetarian diets. *Advances in space research: the official journal of the committee on space research.* 18(4-5): pp. 33-39.

Schab, D. & Trihn, N. (2004). Do artificial food colours promote hyperactivity in children with hyperactive syndromes? A meta-analysis of double blind placebo controlled trials. *Journal of Developmental behaviour paediatrics;* 25: pp 423-34.

Slimak, K.M. (2003). Reduction of autistic traits following dietary intervention and elimination of exposure to environmental substances. *In Proceedings of 2003 International Symposium on indoor air quality and health hazards, National Institute of Environmental Health Science, USA, and Architectural Institute of Japan, January8-11, 2003, Tokyo, Japan, vol 2 pp206-216.*

Shamara, H., Chandola, H.M., Singh, G., Basisht, G. (2007). Utilisation of Ayurveda in health care: an approach for prevention, health promotion, and treatment of disease. Part 1, Ayurveda, the science of life. *Journal of alternative complementary medicine: November 13(9) pp.1011-9.*

Singh, R. H. (2010). Exploring the larger evidence-base for contemporary Ayurveda. *International journal of Ayurveda research: April—June 1(2); pp.65-66.*

Smith, B. (1993). Organic foods vs supermarket foods: element levels. *Journal of Applied Nutrition;* 45: pp.35-39.

Stratham, B. (2002). *The chemical maze.*

Swain, A.R., Soutter, V.L., & Loblay, R.H. (2008). *Friendly foods.* Murdoch Books, NSW.

Swain, A.R. (1988). *The role of natural salicylates in food intolerance.* The University of Sydney.

Swanson, J.M., Sergeant, J., Taylor, E. et al. (1998). Attention deficit hyperactivity disorder and hyperkinetic disorder. *Lancet;* 351: 429-33.

Tapsell, L.C., Hemphill, I., Cobiac, L., Patch, C.S., Sullivan, D.R., Fenech, M., Roodenrys, S., Keogh, J.B., Cliffton, P.M., Williams, P.G., Fazio, V.A., Inge, K.E. (2006). Health benefits of herbs and spices: the past, present and future. *The medical journal of Australia.* Aug; 185(4 Suppl): pp. S4-24.

Trapp, C.B, Barnard, N.D. (2010). Usefulness of vegetarian and vegan diets for treating type 2 diabetes. *Current diabetes reports.* April; 10(2): pp. 152- 158.

Ven Murthy, M.R., Ranjekar, P.K., Ramassamy, C., Deshpande. (2010). Scientific basis for the use of Indian Ayurvedic medicinal plants in the treatment of neurodegenerative disorders. *Central nervous system agentsmedical chemistry; Sept 10 (3): pp238-246.*

Vogtmann, H. (1988). From healthy soil to healthy food: an analysis of the quality of food produced under contrasting agricultural systems. *Nutrition Health;* 6: 21-35.

Wahlqvist, M.L. (1997). Vitamins and vitamin-like compounds. *Allen & Unwin, Australia.*

Walker-Smith, J.A. (1984). Cow's milk protein intolerance in infancy. In *Food intolerance.* Chandra, R.K., (ed). Elsevier, New York.

Welch, A.A., Bingham, S.A., Camus, J., Reeve, J., Day, N., Khaw, K.T. (2005). Calcaneum broadband ultrasound attentuation relates to vegetarian and omnivorous diet differently in men and women: an observation from the European prospective investigation into cancer in Norfolk population study. *Osteoporosis international.* June; 16(6): pp. 590-596.

Welch, A.A., Bingham, S.A., Reeve, J., Khaw, K.T. (2007). More acidic dietary acid-base load is associated with reduced calcaneal broadband attentuation in women but not in men: results from the EPIC-Norfolk cohort study. *The American journal of clinical nutrition.* April; 85(4): pp. 1134—1141.

Wikipedia. (2011). The free encyclopedia. *en.wikipedia.org*

Williams, D. (2008). Living with autism. In *Everyday Health;* 18(3).

Wilson, B. (2008). *Swindled: from poison sweets to counterfeit coffee, the dark history of food cheats.* John Murray, London.

Worthington, V. (2001). Nutritional quality of organic versus conventional fruits, vegetables and grains. *Journal of Alternative and Complementary Medicine;* 7(2): pp. 161-173.

Wynn, E., Krieg, M.A., Lantham-New, S.A., Whittamore, D.R., Burckhardt, P. (2008). Low estimates of dietary acid load are positively associated with bone ultrasound in woman older than 75 years of age with a lifetime fracture. *The journal of nutrition.* July;138(7): pp.1349-1354.

Wynn, E., Krieg, M.A., Lantham-New, S.A., Burckhardt, P. (2010). Postgraduate symposium: positive influence of nutritional alkalinity on bone health. *Proceedings of the nutritional society.* Feb;69(1): pp.166—173.

For more information and updates visit my website www.kyliefloate.com and find me on facebook at my page the undeniable truth about FOOD.